What You
Don't Know
Can Kill
You

What You Don't Know Can Kill You

A Physician's Radical Guide to
Conquering the Obstacles to
Excellent Medical Care

Laura Nathanson, MD

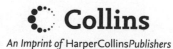

Collins
An Imprint of HarperCollinsPublishers

HarperCollins books may be purchased for educational, business, or sales promotional use. For information, please write: Special Markets Department, HarperCollins Publishers, 10 East 53rd Street, New York, NY 10022.

FIRST EDITION

Designed by Joseph Rutt

Library of Congress Cataloging-in-Publication Data
Nathanson, Laura.
What you don't know can kill you / by Laura Nathanson.—1st ed.
p. cm.
ISBN: 978-0-06-114582-7
ISBN-10: 0-06-114582-3
1. Medical errors—Prevention.   2. Medical care—United States.   3. Patient education.
I. Title.
R729.8.N383 2007   2006051733
610.28'9—dc22

07 08 09 10 11 WBC/RRD 10 9 8 7 6 5 4 3 2 1

I dedicate this book to the memory of my dearest Chuck.

Acknowledgments

I wholeheartedly thank those who have helped with the professional editing and publication of this book: my editor at HarperCollins, Matthew Benjamin, who led me to the right way to tell this story; my very responsive attorney at HarperCollins, Beth Silfin, and the patient folks in Production who put up with so much. Thanks, too, to my agent, Kevan Lyon, and all the folks at the Sandra Dijkstra Literary Agency, who have given me enormous support and encouragement.

I am deeply grateful to all the others who gave so much of themselves to help our family. We were overwhelmed by the kindness and love of family, friends, neighbors, patients, colleagues, and helpers of all descriptions. Chuck's physicians and members of the hospital administration and staff at Vanderbilt, MD Anderson, and UCSD went way, way beyond the extraordinary in their expertise and caring. My legal advice is that I not mention any of you in print, but your names are engraved on my heart. Please, all of you, accept my great thanks and affection. You know who you are.

Contents

Introduction

Our medical care today is famously effective, producing apparent miracles; at the same time, it is notoriously error-prone. I have lived on both sides of this paradox.

Back when I was a pediatric resident, my child patients with the most common kind of leukemia all died; now 95 percent survive. In training, we were told not to try to resuscitate a premature baby of less than thirty-two weeks or under four pounds: now babies of twenty-six weeks and less than two pounds often survive. We used to think X rays and EKGs were pretty snazzy: ultrasounds, CT scans, and MRIs were just a twinkle in their inventors' eyes. Yes, we've come a long way.

But I'm also a bereaved wife. My beloved husband, Chuck Nathanson, age 61, died at home in my arms at dawn on June 5, 2003. A rare tumor of the thymus, a gland above the heart, had first shown itself on his chest X ray in January 2000. The tumor (a thymoma) was the size of a peach, but it went unrecognized by no fewer than six doctors.

A treatable tumor had shown up on an X ray but went undetected for twenty-two months! When I look back on that long period of delayed diagnosis and how we were then and later bounced around from one medical specialist to another, the image that pops into my head is that of a slightly mad, grotesque volleyball game—with the patient as the ball.

There is not much teamwork going on in this game. The player in possession of the ball serves it with little or no expectation that the receiver will acknowledge the serve, much less return it. Sustained volleys are rare. Every now and then a referee from managed care comes through, stops the play, removes some of the players, and replaces them with others. Sometimes the ref picks up the ball and takes it off to a different game in a different part of the park.

Reports from the media suggest that this wacky medical care game is starting to border on anarchy:

- A tumor is missed on the chest X ray *specifically* ordered to check for one, and fifteen months later the world-famous paleontologist Stephen Jay Gould dies of a treatable cancer.

- Someone forgets to take the oxygen tank out of the room before the MRI machine is turned on; the tank becomes magnetized, hurtles around the room, and kills the six-year-old on the table.

- A baby in the neonatal intensive care unit is given breast milk through the tube that enters the vein, rather than through the tube inserted into the stomach, and the baby dies.

- An internist finds a lump in her breast, and her HMO refuses to let her have a mammogram—even if she pays for it herself.

These are not isolated events. Here is the judgment of Donald Berwick, MD, president of the Institute for Healthcare Improvement:

A patient with anything but the simplest needs is traveling a very complicated system across many handoffs and locations and players. And as the machine gets more complicated, there are more ways it can break.[1]

---

1. Quoted in Nancy Gibbs and Amanda Bower, "Q: What Scares Doctors? A: Being the Patient; What Insiders Know About Our Health-Care System That the Rest of Us Need to Learn," *Time* magazine, May 1, 2006, page 44.

Whether you prefer the image of an out-of-control volleyball game or a breakdown-prone machine, today's health care system violates the cardinal rule of effective management: Somebody must be in charge of any complex human system, or it is bound to malfunction.

Medical care today has led to one series of unintended consequences after another. Specialists and scientific discoveries proliferate, bringing with them an enormous need for coordination, interpretation, and above all, leadership in charge of the process. That need has gone unmet. As a result, patients often—and justifiably—feel that "nobody's in charge."

- **Your primary care physician and your specialists aren't in charge.** These hands-on clinical physicians are supposed to suggest possible diagnoses and order studies to arrive at what is called a "definitive diagnosis"—that is, a diagnosis that is not guesswork, but firmly established. If they work in a teaching office, hospital, or clinic, the people who actually do this work may be medical students or doctors-in-training. Their work is supposed to be critiqued by senior physicians.

  When oversights and logical glitches occur, there is no one whose job it is to catch them. Moreover, there is no person or system whose job it is to make sure student doctors' work is truly monitored. The people who commit such glitches are the very least likely ones to be able to spot and correct them. Everyone knows that as individuals we are pretty incapable of spotting our own logical flaws. We wouldn't want to put students in charge of grading their own papers, or scientists to serve as their own peer review. Every published book needs an editor, not just an author.

- **"Data doctors" aren't in charge.** These specialists are supposed to interpret the studies ordered by your clinical physicians. They may have no idea why a particular study was ordered, and may be too rushed to give that question full attention. In the process, errors and oversights occur and are rarely caught by the people who make them.

- **In-hospital physicians aren't in charge.** "Hospitalists" have two conflicting duties: to care for inpatients and to keep the hospital itself running smoothly. Which duty overrides the other may be difficult for anyone, even the hospitalist, to determine.

- **Nurses aren't in charge.** It used to be that nurses protected everyone: young physicians from their own inexperience, seasoned ones from loss of face, and patients from loss of faith. But we are in the midst of a nursing shortage that has amputated that part of the profession.

- **Nobody tells you how to choose the right health care plan.** It is in the interest of the plans that you choose one that is economical *for that plan*. Not the one that is best for you. That is why the plans tell you to start by choosing your primary care provider (PCP). But once you have done so, you have embedded yourself in that particular provider's web of hospitals, specialists, and emergency rooms. That network has been negotiated for the financial benefit of the plan—not for the individual needs of the patient.

That's the bad news.

The good news is that **you** can become the person in charge of your own—or a loved one's—medical safety.

Yes, *you*. I am writing this book to help you avoid what happened to me and to my Chuck. I learned the lesson of the title in the very hardest way. If I had taken the precautions set forth in this book, my husband of thirty years might be with me today.

You won't need any medical training, and I promise not to try to teach you any. All you need is your human intelligence and caring—and a guide. That's my job.

At this time in America, there is only one sure way to safeguard yourself or someone you love. You must be your own fact-checker during the process of diagnosis, your own watchdog during hospitalization, and your own managed care advisor when choosing a health care plan.

Here's what I've learned, and what you must learn if you wish yourself and your loved ones to survive a bout with serious illness. No matter who you are, physician or not, lucky or not; no matter how rich, famous, successful, good-looking, innocent, kindly or powerful; no matter how close and trusting the relationships you have with those providing your medical care—you cannot rely on today's medical system to keep you healthy, safe and alive.

I learned all this the hardest possible way. My great hope is that I can help you, my non-medically-trained readers, to seize hold of your own medical destiny in the interest of preserving your health and your very lives.

PART ONE

The Dicey Diagnosis

ONE

Breaking All the Rules

On May 8, 2002, I found myself in the Patient Services Computer Room of the MD Anderson Cancer Center (MDA) in Houston. Chuck, my beloved husband of 30 years, was ensconced several floors below in the Infusion Center, receiving his third and final course of chemotherapy for a rare, very advanced chest tumor. During the first course, he was too sick for even family to visit. For the second one, his 90-year-old dad, Ben, flew in from Detroit. This time, our daughter Sara had taken off time from Public Defenders in D.C. and was keeping Chuck entertained chatting about her fiancé, fellow law student Joaquin Sanchez.

Chuck and I had been commuting between San Diego and Houston for five months now. This first phase of his treatment—three rounds of high-potency chemotherapy—had gone very well, and had shrunk the tumor considerably. After a rest back in San Diego following this last round of chemo, we'd return in June. At that time, MDA chest surgeons would try to remove every single bit of tumor remaining. Then would come radiation therapy, and finally more chemotherapy to, the oncologists called it, "mop up."

Linda, the MDA Associate Director of Patient Business Services, had waited until our second visit, in March, to broach a delicate subject. I think she had waited until it was clear the chemo was working.

Chuck's care over its entire course, Linda told me, was likely to cost well over $100,000. "*Well* over," she repeated, patting my hand. She was patting my hand because, as she pointed out, our insurance was not required, by contract, to cover *any* of it, not one penny. That's because Chuck and I had broken all the Managed Care rules in getting him to MD Anderson.

Here is why we did so. It is a two-part story.

Part I: On Friday, January 31, 2000, Chuck was diagnosed with fluid around the heart by doctors at our local clinic. He was treated, improved rapidly, and was discharged the next day. Over the ensuing months, he appeared to recover entirely.

Part II: On Sunday, November 4, 2001 (22 months later), his pain and trouble breathing recurred. This time, doctors at the same clinic discovered that he'd had a tumor in his right chest all along, obvious on the chest X ray from January 2000; and that in the interim the tumor had invaded most of Chuck's right lung. After multiple tests, our local doctors told us that they could not identify the source—the kind of tissue composing this particular tumor. Since they couldn't diagnose it, they couldn't treat it. It was, they said, undiagnosable, untreatable, and rapidly fatal. They told us not to make a follow-up appointment until Chuck's symptoms became severe. And by the way, they thought that Vanderbilt Cancer Center in Nashville was doing cutting-edge research on this topic.

We asked our dear friends to help us and in December 2001 we fled, as if pursued by a monster, to Nashville, where Chuck was diagnosed with a rare, advanced, but treatable "malignant thymoma."

Within a week of the diagnosis, other friends helped us get an immediate appointment at MD Anderson where, on January 4, 2002, we learned of their protocol for curing—yes, curing, without recurrence!—advanced thymoma. A week later, Chuck began the long, tough road of chemotherapy, surgery, radiation, and more chemotherapy—a minimum, we were told, of a year's intensive treatment.

Our insurance contract mandated that any out of network care had to be initiated by our San Diego doctors, and pre-authorized by the network itself. Our out-of-state visits were so far out of network, and so unauthorized, we might as well have gone to the moon on our own and expected them to pick up the tab.

Linda assured us that she understood why we had acted so precipitously. But the task at hand was to convince Chuck's insurance company that we had had no choice, that we had had an urgent and compelling need to violate the contract.

She said she thought we might have a chance of getting the insurance company to authorize our out of network flight retroactively. That meant that they would pay 60 percent of the total costs. That would leave Chuck and me with maybe "only" $40,000 to pay out of pocket. Or maybe more. Maybe a whole lot more. Oh, I said.

"It's worth a try," she said, patting my hand again.

I had to agree. So once we were back in San Diego, I went to the clinic and asked for a record release form, which I took home and had Chuck sign. (Since April of 2003, a Federal law called HIPAA has allowed all Americans to obtain and review his or her own medical records. Prior to that, many states insisted that records be transferred only from doctor to doctor.)

I asked for a copy of the entire chart and was presented, the next day, with a four-inch stack of paper bundled into two rubber bands. Flying back to Houston in May of 2002, with Chuck in a Che-Guevara-type gift beret covering his chemo-bald head, both of us in hospital masks, and me lugging a five-pound briefcase, we pretty much became the new best friends of the security officers.

How lucky, we told each other, that our physician and academic friends had gotten us help so quickly! What did people who didn't have such friends do? Or any medical training themselves?

What I now know for certain is that neither dear friends, nor luck, nor money, *nor even medical training*, is what you need to survive the built-in booby traps of our medical care system. What you need is vigilance over your own care as it happens. Because once something dire gets started, all the expertise and goodwill in the world may not be enough to fix it.

TWO

Tracking the Story

- **Find the relevant documents.**

- **Find the relevant section.**

- **Get rid of the "medicalese," the incomprehensible terms.**

According to Linda, our best chance for getting financial help was to write a detailed letter telling not only *what* had happened, but *how* it had happened. How had the tumor been missed in January of 2000? Why hadn't the correct diagnosis been made in November of 2001? What justified our unauthorized flight from San Diego?

To find out how it all happened, and document it, I pulled out the particular chart documents most likely to tell the story.

These documents fall into two groups. The first group is composed of documents produced by clinical care providers—the doctors (and the students, nurses, and residents they supervise) who talk with, examine, and order studies on patients. These documents include hospital admissions, important office visits, and consultations by specialists.

The second group is documents produced by data doctors—the doctors who interpret all those tests ordered by your clinical care providers. You are not likely to meet any of these data providers, as they tend to stay wherever their data is generated—for instance, the radiologists mostly lurk in the X ray department, the echocardiogram-reading cardiologists in the cardiology lab, the biopsy-reading pathologists in the pathology lab.

Happily, all these documents are generally easy to find and, importantly, they are almost always printed rather than handwritten. Either they have been dictated and transcribed, or have been printed out from an electronic medical record, or, rarely, typed by the physician.

All the documents have one thing in common: a section devoted to thinking about the diagnosis. This section can be called Assessment, or Diagnosis, or Problems and Plan, or Impression, or Conclusions, or any synonym thereof.

You probably think that a typical physician interpretation would be a jungle of verbiage, some of it scary and much of it gibberish with lots of syllables. You would be correct.

So your first job is to reduce this hostile prose to something much more reader-friendly. You need to get rid of the unfamiliar terms so that they don't distract you and so that you can focus on the actual thinking process of the writer. I illustrate this pleasing technique below.

CHUCK'S RECORD

The first document I pulled was Chuck's initial encounter with medical care: the Admitting History and Physical Exam on Friday, January 31, 2000.

That winter afternoon, Chuck had made an emergency visit to his internist because of chest pain on his right side and a fever. His doctor thought he was having a gall bladder attack and sent him to the emergency room to be diagnosed.

Chuck called me at my pediatric office. I had never heard his voice like that, full of pain and apprehension. I signed out my patients to my partners, got into my car, and dashed off.

The study—an ultrasound (see the Glossary)—ordered by the emergency room doctor showed that Chuck's gall bladder was fine, but that his heart was big and swollen and that the sac around it was filled with fluid. The emergency room physician immediately transferred Chuck to the cardiology service, and they admitted him to the hospital.

The Admitting History and Physical Exam document from that admission was typewritten and three pages long. I turned to the end, and found the section that revealed the diagnostic reasoning of the physician-author—in this case, it was labeled "PROBLEMS AND PLAN."

Here it is.[2] Don't shake it or you'll get syllables all over yourself.

PROBLEMS AND PLAN:

Incidental pericardial effusion. This patient gives a good story for a pericarditic process progressing to an effusive pericarditis over the last two weeks. Given the timing and the gradual diminishing of his symptoms, this is a good prognosis and indicates most likely that the patient has a viral/idiopathic effusive pericarditis.

However, other more serious etiologies need to be ruled out. I feel a chest X ray to rule out any obvious mass which is evidence against a malignant pericardial effusion. An echocardiograph will of course be obtained to ensure absence of diastolic collapse or any pericardial masses or nodes. Likewise, this echocardiogram will reveal any segmental wall abnormalities which would be evidence against or in favor of a postmyocardial infarction/Dressler syndrome paracentesis/effusion. Other etiologies to entertain would be tuberculosis effusion, which would be assessed by PPD, and viral effusion, most commonly a Coxsackie, which would be assessed by appropriate serologies. His travel to Mexico makes atypical infections slightly higher on the list, but a workup at this time is likely not indicated aside from what I have already mentioned.

At this time, I do not feel a pericardiocentesis is in order; the patient is hemodynamically intact and there is no pulsus paradoxus on further exam. A TSH and ANA will also be obtained in addition to the aforementioned studies. The patient will be admitted and placed on telemetry and in the meantime will be placed on Indocin. If this resolves his

---

2. Document: 1/31/2000, end page 2, top page 3.

symptoms, the patient may be discharged and worked up as an outpatient. We will discuss this with cardiology.

Chuck's Record, Medicalese Removed and Replaced with the Word "Thing"

Now take your pencil and cross out *every medical term* you encounter, anything you don't recognize as ordinary English. Go ahead. Be brutal. For each term you have thus obliterated, substitute the word "Thing" for a noun or verb, "Thingy" for an adjective, and "Thingally" for an adverb. (Exception: there is one word that is medicalese but which needs to stay. That word is "etiology." It simply means "cause." So you can draw a line through it, but then pencil in "cause" above it.)

PROBLEMS AND PLAN:

1. THING. This patient gives a good story for a THINGY process progressing to a[n] THING over the last two weeks. Given the timing and the gradual diminishing of his symptoms, this is a good prognosis and indicates most likely that the patient has a THING.

However, other more serious ~~etiologies~~ causes need to be ruled out. I feel a chest X ray to rule out any obvious mass which is evidence against a malignant THING. A[n] THING will of course be obtained to ensure THING. Likewise, this THING will reveal any THING. Other ~~etiologies~~ causes to entertain would be THING which would be assessed by THING and THING. His travel to Mexico makes atypical infections slightly higher on the list, but a workup at this time is likely not indicated aside from what I have already mentioned.

At this time, I do not feel a THING in order; the patient is THING-ALLY intact and there is no THING on further exam. THING will also be obtained in addition to the aforementioned studies. The patient will be admitted and placed on THING and in the meantime will be placed on THING. If this resolves his symptoms, the patient may be discharged and worked up as an outpatient. We will discuss this with cardiology.

Chuck's Record: the Essence

That was better, but fairly weird. We now have some sentences which the use of the word THING renders meaningless. Let's get rid of those. Here's what happens when we do so:

1. This patient gives a good story. Given the timing and the gradual diminishing of his symptoms, this is a good prognosis.

However, other more serious causes need to be ruled out. I feel a chest X ray to rule out any obvious mass which is evidence against a malignant THING. His travel to Mexico makes atypical infections slightly higher on the list, but a workup at this time is likely not indicated aside from what I have already mentioned.

If this resolves his symptoms, the patient may be discharged and worked up as an outpatient. We will discuss this with cardiology.

There. We can now move to the next chapter, and to the search for "red flags" in this document. A red flag is anything that raises a potentially dangerous problem for the patient.

THREE

Red Flags:
Physician Narratives

Hunt for the three red flags:

- **Scary words and terms**

- **Uncertainty indicators**

- **Fuzzy logic**

Figure out if the diagnosis is certain or up in the air.
If it is up in the air, keep at it until you get it defined.

This simplified "thinking section" of the narrative is now ready for us to inspect for red flags. There are three kinds of red flags: a scary word or term; a word or term or phrase that suggests an uncertain fact or diagnosis; and fuzzy logic, in which there is a flaw in physician reasoning and/or expression.

SCARY WORDS AND TERMS

Most scary words in a medical report are ordinary terrible words, familiar and easy to spot; for instance: *malignant, cancer, brain damage, amputation, dire prognosis, deformity, paralysis, collapse, untreatable, incurable, degeneration, dementia, coma.* Some are phrases: anything beginning with the word "overwhelming" or "irreversible" is likely to be scary. The word "abnormal" should be regarded as scary until you determine exactly what is being so described.

Specific, well-known diseases are also scary words. Cancer, leukemia, cystic fibrosis, and meningitis are examples. Do you need to worry you'll miss a scary diagnosis because you don't recognize a specific disease as scary? No. It would be rare for one of them to appear in a report without other scary words to alert you.

Other words are scary only when used medically. Take "mass," for instance. In ordinary speech, it just means "lump" (unless it has a religious meaning), and is neither scary nor reassuring. But when used in a medical report, read it as "malignant lump" or "cancer." "Mass" is a scary word until proven otherwise.

Another such word is the word "lesion." Lesion is a word that physicians have come up with to describe "something I can see or feel." It could be a spot on your cheek, a lump in your tongue, a shadow on an X ray. Mosquito bites can be called "lesions." So can zits. So can a suspected tumor. For our purposes, regard "lesion" as a scary word until proven otherwise.

SCARY WORD	ENGLISH TRANSLATION
• Benign	Not cancer or not the dangerous form
• Etiology	Cause
• Functional	Normal
• Gross	Big or large or large amount
• Grossly	How it appears to the naked eye, as in "grossly normal"
• Lesion	Possible cancer

SCARY WORD	ENGLISH TRANSLATION *(continued)*
• Mass	Possible cancer
• Metastasis	Spread of cancer
• Negative	Normal
• Pathologic	Abnormal
• Positive	Abnormal, unless it describes a pregnancy test, in which case substitute pregnant
• Septic	Overwhelmingly infected
• Toxic	Dangerously ill
• Unremarkable	Seems normal

UNCERTAINTY INDICATORS

If you have found something that is scary, the next step is to figure out whether this is a definitive, proven diagnosis, or just a possible one in a list of several other possible diagnoses. See Glossary entry for "Diagnosis."

Scary Diagnosis: Definitive

A definitive diagnosis is one that a physician is convinced is the explanation for an illness. For a diagnosis to be truly definitive, it has to be proven by a specific test that is *only* and *always* positive when that diagnosis is the correct one. For instance, an extra chromosome predicts abnormality in the fetus; a "sweat test" is positive for cystic fibrosis; a biopsy shows a specific type of cancer.

If the physician has given a *definitive* diagnosis that is scary, you might think "Well, that is that, there is no reason to pursue it any further." This is not the case. Most of the time a scary definitive diagnosis is correct. *But not all the time.*

- Even a "definitive" test may give a false positive. An extra chromosome from a fetus in the womb, for instance, may have resulted from testing only a small number of cells, whereas it turns out that the overwhelming number of cells in the baby are normal. This is called "mosaicism."

- What appears to be a definitive test may, in fact, not be. Many physicians regard a positive sweat chloride test as the definitive test for the disease cystic fibrosis, but there are at least nine other possible causes, including malnutrition and poor testing technique.

- There are many reports of mislabeled specimens (the wrong patient's biopsy or lab test):

Diagnosed with a deadly . . . cancer at age 34, Kim Tutt was told she might have just months to live. After five surgeries to . . . remove her lower jaw and teeth, and reconstruct her face with bone taken from her lower leg, . . . the mother of two heard some shocking news: The slides from the biopsy . . . had been contaminated by cells from another patient, and she had never had cancer in the first place.[3]

I urge anyone with a scary, definitive diagnosis to obtain a second opinion on whether further tests are needed. The second opinion physician ideally should be a recognized expert in the field. See Appendix for guidance in finding one.

---

3. Laura Landro, "Hospitals move to cut dangerous lab errors," *Wall Street Journal*, June 14, 2006, page D1.

Scary Diagnosis: Not Definitive

A diagnosis that is not definitive is one that is made by excluding other possibilities. Every scary possibility suggested by any physician consulting on the case must be tracked until it is either definitely ruled out or definitively proved. No scary diagnosis should simply be mentioned; each should be fully explored.

The Process of Ruling Things Out

How can you tell if a scary diagnosis is a possibility that has not been either proved or disproved? Check for signs that the physician(s) regard it as an issue not yet settled. I always start by looking for "terms of uncertainty."

Most terms of uncertainty are ordinary words and phrases that bespeak doubt, hesitation, or ambivalence on the part of the writer. For instance: *however, nevertheless, likely and unlikely, most (or less) likely, incidental or coincidental, unclear, less clear, apparently, despite the fact that, uncertain, need to exclude, doubtful or dubious, must rule out, possible/possibility, probable/probability, I feel, I believe, it is my feeling/impression that, evidence for (or against). Given [this], it appears, or gives a good story for.*

But some of the most important words that signify doubt come disguised as technical jargon. Uncertainty can hide in the very stating of the diagnosis! Watch for these hidden-uncertainty terms:

- Idiopathic (nobody knows what causes it)

- Unknown etiology (nobody knows what causes it)

- Unknown primary site (nobody knows where it started)

- Diagnosis of exclusion (we ruled out everything else we could think of, so we figure it's probably this)

- "Probable" anything, as in probable viral infection, probable reactive lymph node, probable innocent murmur (again, we don't know but we figure it's probably this)

- A question mark (?) preceding any term (my best guess, I guess)

If a scary possibility needs to be ruled out, what is the plan to do so? What study, blood test, biopsy, or other procedure is ordered?

"Preshrinking" the thinking portion of the physician's narrative makes the train of thought clear, not clouded with jargon.

Any scary possibility will still be present, and any terms of uncertainty. The thoughtful physician who generates these terms should then give a clear plan to eliminate uncertainty and to try to rule out the scary possibility: a "Rule-Out Plan." If there is no such plan, or if it is not presented in a clear statement, that is the time to address it with your physician.

What is the outcome of the Rule-Out Plan?

Keep tracking this down. Most often, the Rule-Out Plan will involve one or more studies, and thus the participation of one of the data doctors. Data doctors do not treat patients and do not make decisions about them; they don't order tests, medications, diet, etc. Instead, they are experts in "reading" the output of a specific kind of study: biopsies, imaging studies such as X rays or MRIs, EEGs (brain wave recordings), or recordings and images of the heart, and so on.

That reading is dictated (usually) and is part of the medical record. Ideally, you should get hold of every data interpretation as soon as it is available. In the next two chapters, we'll learn how to find red flags in the readings of imaging studies and biopsy reports.

CHUCK'S RECORD

Here is the pre-shrunk version of the "Problems and Plan" section of Chuck's admission on January 31, 2000. I have put the scary and uncertain terms in bold type.

1. This patient gives a good story. Given the timing and the gradual diminishing of his symptoms, this is a good prognosis.

However, other more serious causes **need to be ruled out**. I feel a chest X ray to rule out any obvious **mass** which is **evidence against** a **malignant** THING. His travel to Mexico makes atypical infections slightly higher on the list, but a workup at this time is **likely not indicated** aside from what I have already mentioned.

If this resolves his symptoms, the patient may be discharged and worked up as an outpatient. We will discuss this with cardiology.

There is definitely a scary possibility here: a "**malignant** thing" or a "**mass**."

Has it been excluded with certainty? If not, is there a plan to do so? The sentences telling us that are the following: "**However**, other more serious causes **need to be ruled out. I feel** a chest X ray to **rule out** any obvious mass which is **evidence against** a malignant thing."

Having read these sentences, we still can't tell if a malignant thing, or mass, has been excluded, or if there is a clear plan to do so. This is a fuzzy logic statement.

FUZZY LOGIC

Fuzzy logic can occur in many different forms, in sentences or full paragraphs. Suspect fuzzy logic when something interrupts your sense of the meaning of a paragraph. You may notice this particularly if someone reads the paragraph out loud. You may find yourself raising an eyebrow and saying, "What was *that*?"

To check whether it is truly fuzzy logic, take a pen in hand and write as many versions of the sentence that occur to you and that cannot be clarified by rereading the original. In the following, I have italicized the words I had to add to create all possible meanings I could think of for the sentence:

Fuzzy Logic Sentence

I feel a chest X ray to rule out any obvious mass which is evidence against a malignant thing.

Possible meanings:

I feel *that* a chest X ray *has ruled out* any obvious mass, which is evidence against a malignant thing.

I feel a chest X ray has *not* ruled out any obvious mass, *but if it had, that would be* evidence against a malignant thing.

I feel a chest X ray *should be ordered* to rule out any obvious mass which *would be* evidence against a malignant thing.

I feel a chest X ray *would rule out* any obvious mass, which *would be* evidence against a malignant thing.

So *is* there a chest X ray, and if there is, has it ruled out any obvious mass? Impossible to guess.

This means that until we get further evidence, we are operating under the assumption that a scary possibility exists that has not been either confirmed or ruled out. The scary possibility is a "malignant thing." The apparent way to rule it out is with a chest X ray.

If I had read Chuck's admission history and physical as soon as it was available, I would have spotted the fuzzy logic. My next step would have been either to talk with his cardiologist or to obtain the report of the chest X ray myself, and see what the radiologist really said.

MORAL OF THE STORY

Once you have located fuzzy logic, make sure it is promptly resolved. Fuzzy logic can obliterate a real and dangerous possibility so effectively it never appears again in the chart, and never is evaluated.

FOUR

Red Flags:
Radiology Reports

When we move from the "Problems and Plan" section of the admitting note to the chest X ray report, we move from the clinical care physician to the data doctor.

Clinical care doctors focus on finding out what is going on with the patient. They order studies, whether X rays, lab work, biopsies, or whatever, to clarify the patient's diagnosis and progress. Data doctors focus on interpreting those images, slides, electrical patterns, and so on—they study the studies, and send the results to the clinical care doctors.

The kind of data doctor that is the subject of this chapter is a diagnostic radiologist, a Fellow of the American College of Radiology.[4]

By the time a diagnostic radiologist is credentialed (by the American College of Radiology or by the American Osteopathic Board of Radiology) he or she has been through four years of medical school (MD) or osteopathic school (DO) *plus* five years of postgraduate training (residency). The first year of residency is a preliminary year as a clinical care

---

4. There are two kinds of Fellows in medicine. One kind of Fellow is a physician training for subspecialty program. The other kind of Fellow designates membership of a board certified specialist in that specialty's professional society. For instance, about a million years ago I was a hardworking, sleepless Fellow in the subspecialty of neonatology at Children's Hospital in Detroit. I am today a Fellow of the American Academy of Pediatrics ("Laura Nathanson, MD, FAAP.").

doctor in medicine, surgery, or both. The next four years are in a radiology residency. To become a fully certified radiologist, the resident must pass two written examinations and one oral.

If he nonetheless yearns for more study, apprenticeship, and testing, the credentialed radiologist can then go on to a one- to-two year training in a radiology subspecialty, such as MRI reading, pediatric radiology, or other very focused fields.

You'd think all this would earn board certified radiologists a leisurely, well-paid position in a comfortable work environment. Don't count on it. There are problems in several areas.

THE PROBLEM FOR RADIOLOGISTS

Imaging studies are wonderful. They are almost always virtually painless (at most, a tiny needle prick), safe (if there is any radiation exposure, it is very low; and if general anesthesia is required, it is light and brief), and revealing. Almost any problem in any body part lends itself to an imaging study. For this reason, clinical doctors order scads and scads of them. Scads and scads and scads of them!

No wonder there aren't enough credentialed radiologists to staff all the hospitals in need of them, and to interpret the studies with the care they deserve.

Even if there were, hospitals often feel that they can't afford as many radiologists as they need. Some hospitals outsource some of their readings electronically and cheaply to other countries, especially India. Many hospitals and private radiology groups try to solve the problem by requiring their physicians to work faster and faster. The great thing about employing data doctors is that you can actually count how many studies they read, and set a quota. As a result, the pace is incredible, which is bad for you as a patient, as well for the radiologist.

Thus, the life of a radiologist is often extremely stressful and mole-like. Imagine: There you are in a darkened room, almost always in the chilly dank basement of the hospital,[5] sitting hour after hour, viewing study after study against a brightly lit background, at a breakneck pace, dictating (gabbling!) your findings into the mike even as you turn to the next study. Usually at least one other radiologist is there, similarly occupied, but there's no time for small talk or even for a quick second opinion: "Hey, look at that thing up this kid's nose—I think it's a lapel pin for the Masons!" You can't even chew gum; at the rate you're talking, you'd swallow it.

When you finally finish your day's work, you rise creakily from your chair and leave, blinking in the suddenly glaring lights of the rather dim hallway.

On top of everything else, imaging techniques become obsolete almost as rapidly as cell phones, and radiologists constantly need to update their skills—or manage as best they can with their old ones.

RED FLAGS IN RADIOLOGY REPORTS:
AN ADDED CRUCIAL STEP

The only radiologist who double-checks a radiology report is the radiologist who wrote it. There is nobody in charge of reviewing reports for completeness, much less for accuracy and clarity of expression. One exception: there are institutions that have installed special software with templates that require the radiologist to fill in every item recommended by the guidelines of the American College of Radiology. If one stays blank, the report can't be signed out *or billed for*.

But, you might say, the clinical physician who ordered the report and

---

5. Radiology departments tend towards basements because the equipment requires very cold ambient temperatures and is extremely heavy. Also, the walls and ceilings must be very thick. After all, this is radiation we are dealing with here, and radioactive materials.

receives the interpretation must review it for clarity and completeness. Right? Isn't there a double-check on the report?

Alas, nobody checks that the clinical physician actually does read the report. Every time there is a communication between doctor and doctor, about anything, there is a new opportunity for error. So you, Vigilant One, need to keep a special eye on data reports of all kinds, including radiology reports. Here's how:

First, once again, you preshrink the report:

- Substitute every medical jargon word with "thing," "thingy," etc.

- Search for scary words and uncertain terms.

- See if there is a scary diagnosis that has not been excluded.

- Look for any signs of fuzzy logic.

Then—and this is new—you go on to an additional set of red flags reserved for data reports.

First, the clinical physician has ordered a study to answer a specific question: What's that metallic thing up the kid's nose? Is this wrist fractured? Does this woman have pneumonia? A red flag is indicated by a report's failure to include any of the following:

- The data doctor must make clear that he understands the question—the reason for the test.

- The data doctor must describe his findings clearly enough so that the clinical physician can judge the reasonableness of the data doctor's diagnosis.

- The data doctor also ought to give either a specific diagnosis

("Mason lapel pin high in left nostril") or a differential diagnosis ("Foreign body, metallic, high in left nostril? Barbie slipper charm? earring? part of dog collar?")

- Finally, if the data doctor feels it is appropriate, he should suggest further study or action. ("Recommend prompt removal of foreign body in nose due to danger of aspiration during sniffing.")

The clinical physician and data doctor should be engaged in an active written dialogue where each listens to and queries the other with attention and respect. This means that the clinical physician should review each data report critically to make sure that the most important question has been understood and answered.

The second step in checking a data report is to make sure that its import actually got through to the clinical physician. If a serious error or omission in such a report goes unnoticed by the clinical physician, there can be dire results.

You may recall seeing the following news story about the world-famous paleontologist, Stephen Jay Gould, from an Associated Press release, May 20, 2005. Professor Gould had survived one cancer twenty years earlier, which put him at risk for developing other cancers. So he had frequent check-ups, including chest X rays.

   The family of the late paleontologist and evolutionary scientist Stephen Jay Gould sued two Boston hospitals and three doctors Friday, alleging the famed author would still be alive if they had properly diagnosed his cancer four years ago.
   The doctors all failed to recognize a 1-centimeter (size of a marble) lung lesion on a chest X ray taken of the Harvard University professor in February 2001, according to Alex MacDonald, the lawyer for Gould's survivors.
   Thirteen months later, after another chest X ray was taken, the

lesion had grown to 3 centimeters and the cancer had spread to
Gould's brain, liver and spleen, MacDonald said.

"All of a sudden, it was like out of the head of Zeus, he's got fourth-
stage cancer," Gould's wife, Rhonda Roland Shearer, said in television
interviews on Friday.

Gould, 60, died 10 weeks later, in May 2002.[6]

How could such a thing happen, when the patient was a celebrity, his
physicians alert for exactly such a finding, and the institutions so august? Note that there are three possible explanations for such a disaster:

1. The radiologist did not notice the tumor on the first chest X ray.

2. The report was ambiguous or incomplete, and the clinical
   physician did not clarify it.

3. The radiologist identified the tumor and wrote a full report, but
   the clinical physician either didn't read the report or misread it.

THE NEW RED FLAG FOR DATA REPORTS

The last two explanations for error are ones that you, and only you, can
find and correct before it's too late. Once an incorrect data report is rati-
fied as "not worrisome" by a clinical care physician, it is very unlikely to
be corrected by anyone else.

Here, then, is the new red flag that should arouse your utmost vigilance:

• Make sure the radiologist's report clearly states what he is
  supposed to look for.

---

6. Mark Pratt, "Family of Stephen Jay Gould files wrongful death lawsuit," Associated Press, May
20, 2005.

- Make sure the report clearly states whether or not he found it.

- Make sure that the evaluation clearly states whether the finding is definite and unambiguous.

If any of these three steps is missing, that red flag can spell big trouble.

Chuck's X Ray Report

With this in mind, here is the reading of Chuck's chest X ray report of January 31, 2000.[7] This is the chest X ray that showed the original tumor, as pointed out by the emergency room physician twenty-two months later. Bear in mind that the big question this report is supposed to answer, according to the Cardiology Admitting Report: Is there "any obvious mass" that might indicate a "malignant thing?"

> Charles E. Nathanson
> 1/31/2000 5:45 PM—GD CHEST AP/PA LAT
> TECHNIQUE: [plain chest X ray]
> HISTORY: Epigastric pain
> REFERENCE: None [No previous films for comparison]
> *FINDINGS*: PA and lateral view of the chest reveal extreme cardiomegaly with configuration most likely representing a pericardial effusion. There is prominence of the azygos vein and some earlier cephalization of flow. The lungs are clear. However, there is pleural thickening along the right mid thorax laterally overlying the 6th and 7th ribs.
> IMPRESSION:
> High probability of pericardial effusion.
> Pleural thickening right mid chest laterally.
> Comment: the case was discussed with [*the emergency room physician who admitted Chuck to Cardiology*] at the time of interpretation.

---

7. "Final Report Electronic Signature" 1/31/2000.

First, of course, we substitute all medical terms with the words "thing" or "thingy."

TECHNIQUE:
HISTORY: Thingy pain
REFERENCE: None
FINDINGS: Thingy views of the chest reveal extreme thingy with thingy. There is prominence of the thingy and some earlier thingization of flow. The lungs are clear. However, there is thingy thickening along the right mid thing laterally overlying the 6th and 7th ribs.
IMPRESSION:
High probability of thingy
Thingy thickening right mid chest laterally.
Comment: the case was discussed with [*the emergency room physician*] at the time of interpretation.

Removing all sentences rendered nonsensical by thingies, we get:

TECHNIQUE:
HISTORY: Pain
REFERENCE: None
FINDINGS: The lungs are clear. However, there is thickening along the right mid laterally overlying the 6th and 7th ribs.
IMPRESSION:
thickening right mid chest laterally.
Comment: the case was discussed with [*the emergency room physician*] at the time of interpretation.

CHECKING FOR TWO SETS OF RED FLAGS

First Set: Scary Words, Uncertainty, Fuzzy Logic

Look for Scary Words; if you find any, look for expressions of uncertainty. Conclusion: There are no scary words and no terms of uncertainty.

Is this, then, a reassuring report? Absolutely not. Of course, *you* know that the reason for the study was to "rule out any obvious mass." Or to show any "evidence of malignancy."

So there *should* be a scary word or words in this report, saying that either there is or there is not such a mass/such evidence.

But what if you did not know that? What if the chest X ray had been taken only for routine reasons, such as employment? Would you pass on it as a reassuring examination? No.

Here is the Red Flag: *"The lungs are clear. However, there is thickening along the right mid laterally overlying the 6th and 7th ribs."* Fuzzy logic strikes again! How many ways can these two sentences be written?

The lungs are clear and there is *normal* thickening along the right.

The lungs are clear. However, there is *abnormal* thickening along the right.

There is no way that both of these versions can be correct.

Second Set of Red Flags: Adequacy

The purpose of the second set of red flags is to protect you from overlooking the most serious problem in a data report: ambiguity. A red flag is indicated by the failure of the report to include any of the following:

- Has the clinical physician ordered the study to answer a specific question? Conclusion: There is no specific question—only a symptom: "thingy pain."

- Does the data doctor make clear that the question is understood? Conclusion: There is no such clarification.

- Does the data doctor give a clear description of his findings? Conclusion: No.

- The data doctor ought to give either a definitive diagnosis or a differential diagnosis. Conclusion: Not done. The "Impression" is exactly the same as the "Findings."

- Finally, if the data doctor feels it is appropriate, he should suggest further study or action. Conclusion: Not done.

You see here overwhelming evidence of the reddest of red flags: The report contains fuzzy logic and is remarkably incomplete.

MORAL OF THE STORY

Above, I said that there were three possible explanations for Professor Gould's missed tumor on X ray:

- The radiologist did not notice the tumor.

- The report itself was ambiguous or incomplete, and the clinical physician did not clarify it.

- The radiologist identified the problem correctly and wrote a full report, but the clinical physician either didn't read the report or misread it as normal.

In the case of Professor Gould, we don't know which of the three scenarios applies. In Chuck's case, however, we do know that at least two occurred. We have red flags on its failure to meet the standards of an adequate data report. The clinical physician who wrote the admission history and physical mirrored that incompleteness and ambiguity in the fuzzy logic statement.

If Chuck's chest X ray report had been complete and unambiguous, it would have looked something like this. I have clarified some of the medical terms, using brackets.

Corrected Version of Chuck's X Ray Report

Charles E. Nathanson

Chest X ray 01/31/2000:

HISTORY: Epigastric [above the belly button] pain, seen in ER and Gall Bladder Ultrasound obtained there.

REFERENCE: Ultrasound showed negative gall bladder but large pericardial effusion [amount of fluid in sac around the heart]. There are no previous chest X rays for comparison.

FINDINGS: Extreme cardiomegaly [very enlarged heart] with configuration suggesting pericardial effusion [fluid in sac of heart] as per Ultrasound. The lungs are clear. However, a right sided pleural [lining of the lung] mass is noted, approximately 3.5 cm at largest dimension, along the lateral ribs 6 and 7.

LIMITATIONS: Enlarged heart prevents assessment for other possible masses.

IMPRESSION:

Cardiomegaly [enlarged heart], obscuring mediastinal and hilar areas [lung and chest areas close to the heart].

Pericardial effusion confirmed on prior ultrasound.

Mass lateral right pleura [lining of the lung], assumed to be new.

DIFFERENTIAL DIAGNOSIS: Malignancy most likely cause of mass and possible cause of pericardial effusion [fluid around heart].

FOLLOW UP STUDIES: Chest CT, sample of fluid, obtained under ultrasound guidance, for pathology analysis.

This is the minimum requisite quality of completeness and clarity that should be expected both by vigilant laypersons and by clinical physicians.

Up in the MD Anderson Patient Computer Room, I sat there, wondering how I was ever going to come to terms with this discovery. If I had seen this X ray report in February 2000, Chuck would have had all the benefits of prompt diagnosis and treatment.

We were both paying for my blind trust and lack of vigilance. Stephen Jay Gould's widow and I find ourselves in the same sad situation. I am writing this book to prevent you from joining us.

FIVE

Red Flags:
Medical Volleyball

At this point, I knew two things to put in my insurance letter. First, Chuck's chest X ray of January 31, 2000 had never really been read. The report lacked every one of the pieces of information it was supposed to provide.

Second, this report was never revealed as inadequate. Instead, the clinical physician who wrote the admitting history and physical transformed a meaningless report into a meaningless sentence of Fuzzy Logic: "However, other more serious etiologies need to be ruled out. I feel a chest X ray to rule out any obvious mass which is evidence against a malignant pericardial effusion."

Was there more to include in the insurance letter? Yes.

MEDICAL VOLLEYBALL

In the Introduction, I likened the relationship between consulting physicians to a slightly mad volleyball game, with the patient as the ball. Each team member has as a goal to get the ball back in play. Once he gets that ball back in play, it is no longer that team member's concern. The back-and-forth one would expect in volleyball, or a medical dialogue, is often missing.

This was reflected not only in the radiology report and admission note, but in Chuck's follow-up care after his hospitalization.

His first visit was on February 9, to the cardiologist who had discharged him from the hospital. The report is very brief, noting that Chuck still had some pain, but with no mention of attempts to pin down the cause of the illness.

By the time February turned to March, Chuck was still having some chest pain. I insisted that he make an appointment with his internist, to make sure that there were no worrisome leftover problems. The visit was for March 6. Chuck told me that the cardiologist had planned blood work for the next visit with him, on March 10. To save time, I drew Chuck's blood myself and brought home the results for him to take to the internist and to the cardiologist. The results were neither scary nor reassuring—slight anemia and signs of persisting infection or inflammation.

Here's how the medical volleyball bounced, as reflected in the physician reports.

On February 9, the cardiologist had written:

Impression: Resolving pericarditis probably viral.
Will continue on his current [medication]. Will check him again in a month. Recheck [blood work].

On March 6, Chuck saw his internist. According to her own report, she did not consult the hospital records or speak with the cardiologist. There is no mention whatsoever of a chest X ray. All of her information about that illness was gleaned from Chuck himself, despite the fact that all the clinical and data reports had been sent to her. On the other hand, she does note that Chuck's blood tests are abnormal, and she seems to be unconvinced that the diagnosis is correct:

ASSESSMENT:
Recent pericarditis, (?) idiopathic.
PLAN: Recheck complete blood count. He has follow up with [cardiologist] planned for next week and will keep that appointment.[8]

---

8. History & physical, date of service not noted but transcribed 03/06/2000.

The term "idiopathic" means "unable to define the cause." What, then, does it mean when there is a question mark before the word idiopathic? I guess it means, "I don't know whether the cause is able to be defined." But when the question mark is in parentheses? Does that mean "I *really* don't know whether this is able to be defined?" or "I think that I don't know, but maybe I do?"

In any event, the only action the internist took was to pop the ball back to the cardiologist.

On March 10, Chuck had his appointment with the cardiologist. At this visit,[9] no procedure (such as an ultrasound of the heart) was performed. The cardiologist does not mention the internist visit; the previous abnormal lab tests I had drawn; the fact that the internist ordered *more* tests for the cardiologist to check at this visit; or even the fact that the month before the cardiologist himself had planned to repeat the blood tests at this visit.

Instead, the cardiologist discharged Chuck from follow-up.

The Volleyball (Chuck) has received its final serve way out of the court. Game over!

THE MORAL OF THE STORY

Never underestimate how intimidated patients can be by physicians. But that's not the only reason patients and those who love them are reluctant to ask questions. Here was Chuck, married to a doctor for thirty years; he might have been expected to make more of a fuss. He could have asked the internist to take more of an interest in the cause of his illness. Certainly one would think that at the very least he would have asked the cardiologist about the blood tests.

Chuck never had trouble asking anybody uncomfortable questions. In fact, that was his job: He had worked for the notoriously inquisitive

---

9. Progress note, 3/10/2000.

Izzy Stone on the famous independent *I.F. Stone's Weekly*; as city editor on the *Detroit Free Press*; and for a decade as director of the San Diego Dialogue, a cross-border University-sponsored problem-solving group— you can just imagine the uncomfortable questions *that* endeavor generated. Chuck was always telling his staff, "Ask questions! The world's at the tip of your tongue!"

So I don't think Chuck was intimidated by his physicians. I think he just didn't want to "push his luck." At one point during his recovery, that spring of 2000, he said to me out of the blue, "I hope that thing doesn't come back to bite us." And that's one reason why I didn't quiz Chuck or his doctors. I hoped so, too. It took nearly two years, but "That Thing" came back and bit with a vengeance.

═══════

SIX

The Monster

From the spring of 2000 to the autumn of 2001, Chuck and I lived without a shadow on our lives. He had a bit less energy than before, and needed a weekend nap—but after all, he was almost 60. We took up dancing lessons in hopes of progressing beyond the basic foxtrot, and at one point had achieved the ability to dance a cha-cha but not, alas, the ability to recognize when a cha-cha was actually being played.

We hiked a lot. In June 2000, we went to Sara's graduation from law school, and bought our newly minted Washington, D.C., public defender a two-compartment briefcase for Christmas. "Oh good," she said, "I'll use one side for drug cases and the other one for homicides." It went right to a parent's heart.

We hiked in Utah and Sedona, and every Sunday ran with our friend Jack through the hills of Torrey Pines State Park, in the cliffs overlooking the Pacific. On September 11, 2001, the phone woke us at 6:00 A.M. with the news that Sara was "all right" but that she was just leaving the federal courthouse because the Pentagon, across the street, and the World Trade Center had been bombed. Neither Chuck nor I was able to stay glued to the TV all day—we had to work—but we were as shaken as if we had been.

A week later, all the hospitals in San Diego began holding doctor classes on bioterrorism: smallpox, anthrax, botulism, plague, nerve gas. My colleagues at El Camino Pediatrics and I quizzed each other and posted informative posters on our bulletin boards. We gently fended off people asking for Cipro prescriptions in case they were exposed to anthrax.

On Sunday, November 4, Chuck had a relapse of the same symptoms—fever, right chest pain, shortness of breath—that had led to his earlier urgent visit on January 31, 2000. Since this was a Sunday, we went to the emergency room without first calling his internist.

There we discovered that we were facing a monster. It stared back at us from the X ray ordered by the young, appalled emergency room doctor.

While Chuck's heart was now perfectly normal in size, big lumpy tumor tissue engulfed his right lung and the area above the heart that doctors refer to as the "anterior mediastinum."

We had our very own bioterrorist.

Our energetic young emergency room doctor ran off to the radiology department and brought back the chest X ray taken 22 months earlier. It was the first time we had seen it. There, a big nasty surprise to all of us, was a mass in the lining of the right lung. It was obvious—about the size of a peach. Our emergency room doctor, highlighting the "peach" with pen markings, wondered out loud whether the very enlarged heart on that first X ray might have hidden some of the tumors now evident in the anterior mediastinum and elsewhere.

He arranged for Chuck to see a lung specialist—a pulmonologist. Over the next few anxious weeks, Chuck underwent a series of tests to see what kind of tumor we were dealing with. His doctors were convinced that the tumor had started in some other part of the body and spread (metastasized) to the right lung and the mediastinum, but all the tests on the rest of him came back normal.

Since she couldn't find the origin of this tumor with blood tests, imaging studies, or direct examination of the intestine, the pulmonologist performed a biopsy of the mass. She used a fine needle under the guidance of a CT scan to help find the tumor. Finally, on November 26, we had an appointment with a physician in the clinic's oncology (cancer) center to tell us the results of the biopsy and to give us Chuck's diagnosis.

A younger doctor took a history from Chuck and briefly examined him. Then the senior doctor walked in and without preamble, and without sitting down, gave us the bad news.

Chuck, he informed us, had CUPS, Cancer of Unknown Primary Site. The tumors in the chest had come from a source other than the lung itself, but from where, it was impossible to tell. The hunt for a primary site—the blood tests and imaging studies—showed all the possible culprits to be innocent. The biopsy had now confirmed this. No matter what organ the pathologist looked for, it wasn't the primary site.

If you don't know the origin of the cancer, the oncology doctor pointed out, you cannot treat it.

There was no treatment for CUPS that was effective, he went on. Most patients with CUPS, he said, die three to four months after diagnosis. In fact, he told us, there was no point in our making a follow-up appointment until Chuck's symptoms became worse; a follow-up visit would be a waste of time. And by the way, researchers at Vanderbilt University, in Nashville, were said to be doing cutting-edge work on CUPS.

He finished and stood looking down at us.

I asked the doctor about the relevance of Chuck's past history—the mass on the X ray nearly two years earlier. He used body language to signify that the matter was irrelevant.

I then asked for a referral for a second opinion to a cancer center (meaning a National Cancer Institute–designated center). The physician replied, "This *is* a cancer center."

He turned and left the room.

"Jerk," said Chuck, to his retreating back. That was strong language for him.

Once again, I did not obtain and review Chuck's medical records. I was stunned and terrified, and frantic to find a way out. I called my dear friend—my senior resident-in-training, and the matron of honor at our wedding on the roof of Boston City Hospital in 1972—Patricia Temple Gabbe, now a pediatrician at Vanderbilt Medical School. With her husband, Steve Gabbe, the dean of the medical school, she arranged for Chuck to be seen there right away.

I took a six-month leave of absence from my practice. My fellow doctors and all the staff took it like the heroes and true friends I'd always known them to be, with not a moment's hesitation, though the increase in their workload in the dead of winter was severe.

Chuck and I caught practically the next plane to Vanderbilt. He was seen instantly and treated royally. We were told that the biopsy performed in San Diego was not sufficient for diagnosis. So Chuck underwent a second biopsy of the tumor, this one performed under anesthesia by a chest surgeon.

On December 29, 2001, the Vanderbilt oncologist called us at home. Chuck did not have an untreatable, incurable Cancer of Unknown Primary Site.

Instead, he had a treatable, though advanced, malignant thymoma. The thymus gland is located in the anterior mediastinum, just above the heart. It's active in fetal life, helping to form the immune system. By the time a child is about four years old, the thymus has usually shrunk so much, you can't see it on an X ray. Malignant thymoma is the most common tumor of the anterior mediastinum. Chuck's maternal grandmother had died of the same thing, at age 58. But it was not supposed to be a "hereditary" cancer.

We decided to seek treatment closer to home, and with the help of our dear friends here in San Diego, were able to set up an immediate appointment at the MD Anderson Cancer Center in Houston, Texas.

There had been a two-month delay from November 4, 2001, when the San Diego emergency room doctor saw the Monster, to January 4, 2002, when the MD Anderson doctors presented us with a plan of treatment. It was a protocol for this particular kind of advanced thymoma, and they had had success in curing it—without recurrence.

Did those two months make a difference in the size and aggressiveness of the tumor? It's impossible to tell. However, avoidable delay in making a diagnosis should be prevented vigorously. I want to show you two more very crucial Red Flags that may have engendered that delay. They are Red Flags on the biopsy (pathology) report, and Red Flags on physician credentials. Hence, the next two chapters.

SEVEN

Red Flags:
Pathology Reports

The San Diego doctor who told us in November 2001 that Chuck had an undiagnosable, untreatable, rapidly fatal Cancer of Unknown Primary Site based his opinion on the pathologist's reading of the biopsy.

Pathologists often refer to themselves as "the doctor's doctor," because their job is to take into account all the lists of possible diagnoses generated by the clinical physicians and, by examining a biopsy (a sample of fluid or tissue), discover the definitive diagnosis. There is an aura of certainty about a "biopsy proven" diagnosis.

This aura, however, can be deceptive. There are enough false negatives (a cancer or other condition is not diagnosed even though it is present) and false positives (a cancer is diagnosed even though it is not present) to warrant a high level of vigilance.

That's why I want you to know exactly what to watch out for and how to prevent problems. There are three kinds of possible traps: Paperwork, technical, and procedural.

PAPERWORK : MAKE SURE THAT
BIOPSY IS REALLY YOURS!

You may recall this story already quoted from *The Wall Street Journal*, June 14, 2006. I just want to impress it upon your memory.

Diagnosed with a deadly . . . cancer at age 34, Kim Tutt was told she might have just months to live. After five surgeries to excise a cyst under her gum, remove her lower jaw and teeth, and reconstruct her face with bone taken from her lower leg, the . . . mother of two heard some shocking news: The slides from the biopsy of her cyst had been contaminated by cells from another patient, and she had never had cancer in the first place.

Ask the physician who performs your biopsy to show you the pre-labeled specimen containers. Make sure that it is your name on the label. You can also ask the pathologist to make sure that the final slides are properly labeled.

TECHNICAL: MAKE SURE THAT THE SAMPLE TAKEN WAS ADEQUATE

This is one reason it is very important to check the biopsy report itself, and see what the pathologist has to say about the sample quality. There are several kinds of inadequate sampling:

- **Too small a sample.** This is particularly important if the sample was difficult to obtain or if the biopsy was obtained through a "fine needle," which, as you might expect, results in a tiny amount.

- **Too many cells to look at.** A second technical problem can arise if the area of the biopsy is large. With PAP tests for cervical cancer, the whole area of the cervix (about half the size of a woman's fist) is the field from which cells are collected. That's a lot of cells. There are two kinds of preparations of those cells: a regular smear, or a thin smear. Ask your gynecologist whether you should have one, the other, or both—depending on your age and previous history.

- **Too few abnormal cells present.** If the sample consists mostly of surrounding normal tissue, or of scar tissue, the abnormal cells may escape notice.

PROCEDURAL: IF THE PATHOLOGIST DOESN'T KNOW TO LOOK FOR IT, HE WON'T FIND IT EVEN IF IT IS THERE

You need to examine what the pathologist looked for, and make sure that he didn't leave something out of his consideration of possible diagnoses.

Pathologists "read" biopsies by putting biopsy material on slides and staining them. Sometimes the pattern of staining is specific for a certain condition. At other times, the ordinary staining patterns may not give a definite answer. The pathologist then performs immunohistochemical stains to determine exactly what he is dealing with. (Let's call these IHC stains.)

IHC stains are specially created. Instead of relying on whether the stain binds to the physical characteristics of a tissue, IHC cells actually seek out tissue "signatures" by recognizing their particular immune profile. This makes them much more specific than other stains. They can be used singly and in combination to exclude or to point the finger at a very specific type of tissue.

But these IHC stains have two pitfalls: First, they are very expensive, and many insurance companies balk if they think the stains are used unnecessarily. Second, they require a great deal of thought from the pathologist, and a very clear idea of what specific tissue types he wants to exclude or explore.

Most often, the pathologist doesn't have access to, or time to read, the patient's chart and develop his own list of possibilities. He relies on the information given by the clinical doctor who has referred the patient for biopsy. *If the clinical physician does not include a possibility, the pathologist is not likely to test for it.*

Of course, if that clinical doctor hasn't given any list of possibilities, the pathologist must go it alone. That means that he must consider what kind of biopsy he's been given (liver, kidney, whatever) and try to track down the culprit causing the illness. Some pathologists are much more thorough and experienced at this than others. Some will have more time and incentive than others.

This is why it is crucial for you to make sure that the list of possible diagnoses given to the pathologist is complete and clear. It is also why it is crucial that you get the biopsy report and make sure that the pathologist has considered every possibility in that list of potential diagnoses.

To do so, you will need a different red flag technique than those we have used in past chapters. In this situation, do *not* delete medical jargon or replace it with the word "thing." Instead, merely circle or highlight each medical term.

You do not need to have a single clue about what the terms mean. This is simply a game of Match-Them-Up, like mah-jongg tiles.

Start with the Lists of Potential Diagnoses

Chuck had been given two lists of possible diagnoses, one from his clinical physician, the pulmonologist, and the other from the radiologist who performed his CT of the chest. The lists differ from each other.

List of possible diagnoses produced by the pulmonologist, dated November 7, 2001:

> The differential diagnosis obviously would be most concerning for malignancy including malignant mesothelioma. Obviously bronchogenic carcinoma . . . would also be in the differential. . . . The best way to proceed is a CT scan with contrast . . . If it does turn out that there are masses, he will need a biopsy.[10]

---

10. Consultation 11/07/2001, pp. 2 and 3.

Terms circled: malignant mesothelioma; bronchogenic carcinoma. Radiologist's reading the CT of the chest, dated November 9, 2001:

Differential diagnosis includes metastases most likely adenocarcinoma (especially lung), mesothelioma, if patient is known to have asbestos exposure . . . Other considerations are malignant thymoma or lymphoma. Findings recorded on Dr. Pulmonologist's voice mail at the time of this study.[11]

Terms circled: Metastases most likely adenocarcinoma (especially lung), mesothelioma, malignant thymoma, lymphoma.

Have Your List Checked

Before the biopsy is performed, ask the doctor who ordered it to check your list of all suggested possible diagnoses.

In Chuck's case, that list would have included all the following, mentioned by the pulmonologist and the radiologist: malignant mesothelioma, bronchogenic carcinoma, metastases most likely adenocarcinoma (especially lung), mesothelioma, malignant thymoma, lymphoma.

WHAT *DID* THE PATHOLOGIST LOOK FOR?: THE BIOPSY REPORT

Take a look at a biopsy report, and you are likely to be instantly reminded of a Brillo pad. It's clearly got a bunch of strands and a pattern behind it, but you couldn't possibly unravel it, and if you tried you'd get hurt by the abrasive contents.

---

11. CT Scan, 11/09/2001

Three Things to Check

1. **Does the report state accurately what organs or tissues were examined?** If that's not the tissue you thought was being biopsied, you need to tell the physician who ordered the biopsy *right now*.

2. **Does it state that the biopsy sample was adequate?** If it does not state this clearly, ask your clinical physician. Sometimes, as in Chuck's case, the information that the sample may have been inadequate is embedded in medicalese: "small to intermediate size cells present in variable sized groups within a densely sclerotic stroma."[12] A "densely sclerotic stroma" is a fancy term for thick scar tissue.

3. **Did the Pathologist indeed investigate all items on the diagnoses list?** I'm going to list this separately.

Question 3: Was Everything Looked For That Should Have Been Looked For?

Turn to the Comment (Assessment, Differential Diagnosis, whatever the Pathologist calls it) section. Fortunately, your task is relatively easy. Get your list of all suggested possible diagnoses. Then check the "Comment" *only* to see whether the pathologist tested for every one of them.

Here is what Chuck's pathologist tested for:

> The immunohistochemical profile would tend to exclude mesothelioma, primary lung cancer, male breast cancer, and prostate cancer. The upper gastrointestinal tract, pancreas, and hepatobiliary system should be evaluated. In all likelihood, the tumor in the mediastinum and pleura are metastatic.[13]

---

12. Pathology consultation, 11/14/01. "Comment."
13. Ibid

Match the "excluded" terms with the list of all possible diagnoses. What has the pathologist not looked for? Lymphoma—and *malignant thymoma*. These were the two possibilities suggested by the radiologist who read the chest CT.

If you find this kind of discrepancy, ask your clinical physician (either your primary care physician or the specialist ordering the biopsy) to tell you why they were not investigated by the pathologist.

MORAL OF THE STORY

A biopsy report can be very valuable but it is not infallible. Do not hesitate to ask for a second biopsy, not just a second opinion, in any situation in which you suspect a false positive *or* a false negative. Here are a few such indications:

- The biopsy is reported as benign, but the mass keeps growing, or you have a worrisome family history, or you have other symptoms such as fever, pain, weight loss.

- The biopsy is reported as positive for a dire or rare disease.

- The biopsy indicates an illness rare in your age group, sex, ethnic background, or history of exposure to chemicals or radiation.

In Chuck's case, the diagnosis of "Cancer of Unknown Primary Site" was made because the pathologist did not look for the correct site and because the correct diagnosis was never considered by his clinical care doctors.

At this point in my discoveries, I decided to check the credentials of his clinical care doctors.

EIGHT

You Can't Tell the Players Without a Program

We all make assumptions about whom we are dealing with. I assume that the character shrouded in hooded white suit, plastic mask, gloves, boots, and ear-splitting equipment who just showed up in my back yard is from Corky's Pest Control. I sure hope that it is. If it isn't, I sure want to know who it is and why he's there! (I think.)

In a medical context, many of us tend to assume that well-spoken people who seem to "own" their role, speak and act confidently, and receive the respect of those around them, are the grown-ups, professionally speaking. Trust me: it's more complicated than that.

In May 2002, as I finished composing the insurance letter, my last topic was the credentials of the writers of the medical record reports who had been responsible for Chuck's and my dashing around the country to Nashville and Houston.

Here is what I found. After I tell you, I'll tell you how I found it, and how you can do so.

WHODUNIT?

The admitting history from January 31, 2000, contained the fuzzy logic statement: "I feel a chest X ray to rule out any obvious mass which is evidence against a malignant thing." That note was written by a *doctor-in-training*, not by one of the cardiologists. The attending physician, a cardiologist, cosigned the report, without flagging or correcting the fuzzy logic.

While teaching hospitals are usually ideal choices for patients with rare or complex problems, the whole structure must be functioning to make them that ideal choice.

It is natural for a medical student or doctor-in-training to try to write an impressive note, one that dazzles the mentor. It is the job of the mentor—the supervising or attending physician—to guard against being so dazzled that the "most important question" is lost in the shadows.

The cardiologist who discharged Chuck from follow-up without clarifying the chest X ray or abnormal lab results was not a general cardiologist, but director of the Lipid Clinic, specializing in all things having to do with cholesterol. This is a complex field that changes frequently, and the director of such a clinic should be assumed to spend many hours developing and administering programs for diagnosis, monitoring, and treatment—dietary and pharmaceutical. However, in many hospitals *all* the doctors in a specialty rotate "on call" care, taking turns evaluating patients who are admitted to the hospital through the emergency room.

Chuck might have been better served by a general cardiologist or even an internist, someone aware that the chest includes more than just the heart and its lipid-sensitive blood vessels.

Chuck's November 2001 diagnosis of "Cancer of Unknown Primary Site" was given in the opening sentence of a report written by a Fellow in oncology, not yet board certified in the specialty. It is not usual to start out such a consultation with a conclusion but rather to reason one's way to that diagnosis by reviewing all the possibilities that have been considered and rejected.

Fellows in a subspecialty are often burdened by multiple assignments, including research and teaching. The Fellow in this department may have been on a tight time schedule.

At any rate, the report of any doctor-in-training is supposed to be reviewed, critiqued, and co-signed by the attending, Board Certified, physician. In this case, neither the Board Certified attending *nor* the doctor-in-training signed the report.

Moreover, this attending physician was board certified, but not in oncology. He was board certified in the specialty of hematology.[14] Hematology is the study of diseases of the blood. Oncology is the study of solid tumors: lung cancers, breast cancers, and, of course malignant thymomas.

The specialties of hematology and oncology are closely allied, and it is possible for an internist who wants to subspecialize to become board certified in both separately, or in a hybrid of the two.

This particular physician was board certified only in the study of blood disorders. Why was Chuck assigned to him? It might have been that Chuck had to be "worked into" the busy clinic schedule, and so was assigned to the doctor "on call" that day.

Your Checklist for Identifying the Players:

- Ask: are you being assessed by a medical student, a resident, a Fellow, or a senior on-staff physician? They are all supposed to tell you, but you may need to ask. One way to find out, if you're shy about seeming to confront them, is to say that you always like to write thank-you notes, and would like one of their professional cards.

- Check the record to see who *dictated* the report. If there is only one space for a signature, that is the signature of the person who both dictated and "fact checked" his own report, usually a senior physician.

- If there are two spaces for signatures, one is the signature of the person who dictated the report, and the other is the signature of

14. American Board of Medical Specialties Web site. www.abms.org

the more senior person who, in signing, confirms that he did indeed "fact check" the report.

- If the name of the person who dictated a cosigned report is followed by "MD" or "DO," this is a doctor-in-training. If these initials after the name are absent, or different initials are there, the person is not a physician. Do not hesitate to ask what the initials mean. They may refer to nurses, physician assistants, or to categories unique to a particular institution.

- To check further on the credentials of a senior physician, go to the American Board of Medical Specialties at www.abms.org.

  American Board of Medical Specialties
  1007 Church Street, Suite 404
  Evanston, IL 60201–5913

- To verify whether a specific physician is board certified, call (866) ASK-ABMS.

- Finally, to find out what kind of work your physician does when he is not the "doctor on call" accepting new patients, ask for his professional card. Or go to your hospital's Web site.

At that point, I felt that I had written to the insurance company everything I had to say. I sealed and mailed the letter, and hurried back down to the chemotherapy infusion center.

The Medical Professional Ascent

Period of Time	Credential Obtained	Required Preparation	Career Options
1–2 Years	SUBSPECIALTY BOARD CERTIFIED Cardiology, Radiation Oncology, Thoracic surgeon, Neonatology	FELLOWSHIP ↑	Practice Research Teaching
2–7 Years	STATE LICENSE ABMS[15] Certified Primary Specialty[16]	RESIDENCY ↑	Practice Research Teaching
4 years	MD or DO	MEDICAL or OSTEOPATHIC SCHOOL ↑	Unlicensed practice
4 years	Diploma B.A., B.S.	COLLEGE: Pre-Med Program	Medical Writer

MILESTONES:

- Medical/Ostopathic School: Pass tests of National Board of Medical Examiners. Obtain State License.

- Residency: Pass two or more exams administered by Specialty Board

- Fellowship: Pass two or more exams administered by Specialty Board

"Fellow" has two meanings: 1. A specialist who is in training to be a subspecialist; 2. A specialist or subspecialist who belongs to an accredited professional organization, such as the college of radiology or the academy of pediatrics.

15. ABMS American Board of Medical Specialties
16. Primary Specialty: Internal Medicine, General Surgery, Pediatrics, OB-GYN

NINE

Home Again, Hospital Again, Home Again

By April 2002, the tumor had been shrunk enough for Chuck to undergo surgery. The goal was to remove every bit of the monster. Malignant thymomas have only one redeeming feature: at least they do not metastasize (spread to other sites in the body). They set themselves up in the thymus gland, above the heart, and spread only to one or the other lung.

Sara, once again taking time off from Public Defenders, and I sat in the MDA chest surgery visitors' lounge playing endless games of double solitaire, interrupted around hour five by a brief visit from the surgeon. He had discovered that he needed to make an incision through Chuck's back, to get at one remaining tumor mass; and that he might need to put Chuck on heart-lung bypass to do so. "I wouldn't consider it at all except that he's in such great physical shape otherwise. But I want to get it all out." Sara and I both said "Go ahead."

As it turned out, they did not need to do the bypass. Finally, after a total of eight hours, Chuck was wheeled into the recovery room. The highly experienced surgeon told us that this was the most extensive chest surgery he had ever performed.

The surgery was a complete success, but the aftermath was dreadful. Chuck developed one air pocket after another, first in the right lung and then in the healthy left one. Time after time, the lung tissue would tear, allowing air to escape into the chest cavity; these air pockets continued to grow as he breathed, and compressed the healthy lung. The surgeons believed that this was most likely because the surgery had been so extensive.

Each air pocket required the insertion of a tube to release the built-up air, so that the pocket wouldn't inflate like a balloon and compress the normal lung. And each of the tubes had to be attached at all times to a source of suction, either the type built into the wall (like a central vacuum) or a portable machine.

On the other hand, the rest of him was doing well, so well that the surgeons wanted him up and walking to lessen chances of complications such as pneumonia and blood clots. This required a portable suction machine. The two of us must have been a sight to behold: Chuck pushing along a wheeled IV pole that held the very impressive suction pump to which he was attached by a long chest tube, the two of us striding around the ward, and then sneaking off behind the elevator bank for a quick canoodling.

Altogether, Chuck was in the post–chest surgery ICU at MD Anderson for five weeks. Finally, there was only one air pocket left in the "good" lung, and it was so tiny it had not required a tube. The doctors felt we could return to San Diego—but by train. The pressure changes with flying might make the air pocket expand catastrophically.

We hadn't counted on the "reduced circumstances" of Amtrak and the primitive conditions on the train, nor on the frequent holdovers to allow freight trains priority on the track, nor especially on the 5,000-foot altitude change going over the mountains.

Somewhere in Arizona, Chuck casually mentioned to me that he was having trouble breathing. We just stayed quiet and calm for the rest of the long ride home. At the University of California San Diego (UCSD) teaching hospital emergency room, where we had transferred our care, Chuck was diagnosed with an 80 percent collapse of his good left lung.

Then came another three weeks of inpatient stay at UCSD, much like the one at MD Anderson, with one chest tube after another. This time there was no portable giant pump for us to walk around with, but a small battery-operated one that sounded like a leaf blower. Chuck would put the pump on a wheelchair, cover it with two pillows to damp the noise, and up and down the corridors we would stride. When people inquired, Chuck told them with a straight face that he'd been hired to clean the corridor carpets. Sometimes this would trigger an appalled glance, and a more appalled silent conjecture, as the questioner noticed Chuck's chest tube attached to the machine.

Finally the suction could be removed, and Chuck was discharged with a small valved device attached to a short chest tube—a Heimlich valve, with no active suction. When the UCSD surgeon examined him for discharge, he shook his head. "You look like St. Sebastian," he said, "except you're still breathing."

When we returned home, I found the letter from the insurance company. They were going to cover everything 100 percent: Vanderbilt, MD Anderson, and UCSD. And anything we might need from them in the future.

I was relieved, but there was a big stone in my stomach. The little money stone was gone, but the great big monster one remained.

PART TWO

In the Hospital

TEN

The Sensitive Sentinel[17]

In all, Chuck wound up spending a total of sixty-seven days and nights as an inpatient in four different hospitals. With the remarkable support of my colleagues at El Camino Pediatrics, I was able to stay with him the whole time.

Chuck and I had been married for half our lives. Of course, it was clear from the beginning that we would go through this together. We were each other's courage.

I know how rare a privilege this is, and I'm well aware that most of us simply cannot just put life on hold and move into a loved one's hospital room. I would love to be able to say that it isn't really necessary, and that most of the time everything goes smoothly.

But I can't do so. I agree with the words of Dr. Donald Berwick, the president of the Institute for Healthcare Improvement, that I quoted in the introduction: "A patient with anything but the simplest needs is traversing a very complicated system across many handoffs and locations and players. And as the machine gets more complicated, there are more ways it can break." (*Time* magazine, May 1, 2006, p. 44.)

Each of us must make the decision based on our own personal circumstances and responsibilities, and on the situation of the patient and

---

17. **Sentinel** is a term invented by *Time* magazine reporters Nancy Gibbs and Amanda Bower in "Q: What Scares Doctors? A: Being the Patient; What Insiders Know About Our Health-Care System That the Rest of Us Need to Learn," May 1, 2006, page 48.

the hospital. Here are five situations any one of which would push my worry-buttons.

- Awareness that the ward is understaffed

- Eye-witnessing one or more care problems, such as the wrong meal being served or the wrong medication being given

- Patient noncompetent due to age (child or elderly with mental deterioration) or illness (unconscious; heavily sedated)

- Patient has more than two "lines" or "tubes." Two tubes are usually fairly low-maintenance. For instance, one might carry intravenous fluids and meds, and the other might serve for giving oxygen through a mask, collecting urine from a tube in the bladder, or a feeding tube into the stomach. Three or more tubes implies both medical fragility and treatment complexity that increases chance of error.

- Patient has rare or dire condition

In Chuck's case, we had one more worry-button situation: our trust in medical care had been shaken by our previous San Diego experience. I felt I couldn't let him out of my sight for a second. And the more time I spent living on hospital wards, the more alert I became, and the more I realized how many things could go awry, even at the finest institutions.

Once we returned to San Diego and Chuck had to be admitted to UCSD Medical Center, we were helped, again, by friends. In particular, I was blessed: I was given a cosentinel. For ten years, Jack Koerper had joined us each Sunday for a four-mile jog in the Torrey Pines State Park, up and down the cliffs bordering the beach. He had recently retired, and was the first friend I called when Chuck arrived at the UCSD Emergency Room with an 80 percent collapse of his good lung. Jack found us right away and then came every single day, for all the weeks.

Not only did he allow me a couple of hours every afternoon to drive home, exercise, open the mail, and shower; he was a hugely normalizing force, engaging Chuck in their ongoing and highly animated discussion of San Diego politics. He helped Chuck bathe and shave. Most of all, he helped me to behave. I was pretty short-tempered by this time, and at several points Jack had to put a hand on my shoulder and glare at me before I took off the head of the nearest physician, nurse, or administrator.

Without Jack, I suspect I might have lost my privileges to stay in Chuck's room overnight.

THE ROLE OF THE SENTINEL

During each hospitalization, I tried to notice every development, ask questions, and advocate on Chuck's behalf. But there was more to it than that. The key to being a Sentinel, I found, is to try to *normalize* and to *make safe* the patient's immediate environment.

Well.

Normalizing the environment requires the attitude that what is happening is expected and nonthreatening. Making the immediate environment safe, on the other hand, requires the assumption that what is happening may be fraught with danger. Tricky. Very tricky.

Normalizing the Surroundings

Fortunately, the very act of normalizing the environment allows a sentinel to develop the ability to keep it safe. Normalizing involves understanding and getting control of your surroundings, identifying the various people and their roles, and becoming able to predict what is likely to happen next. That's a firm basis for being able to know how to get help, and whom to call. Just knowing where the vomit basins are kept is empowering.

But normalizing goes beyond those basics. The patient is captured in an impersonal institution, surrounded by strangers, at the mercy of pain. The sentinel can create a calm, safe, small "other place" within the great big hospital—a bubble-like space that encapsulates you and the patient, walling out strangeness and stress.

- Consciously speak softly and calmly; sit close, touch, make eye contact.

- If you must ask an anxious question that the patient has not already thought of, do so out of the patient's hearing. ("Do you think he'll need another surgery?" "Do you think she'll need a feeding tube?") If the question is on the patient's mind, encourage the patient to be the one doing the asking.

- Let the patient be the one who talks and gets talked to by the medical personnel. Don't interrupt or intervene or speak for the patient, as if he or she were incompetent (unless, of course, that is the case). I remember one time Chuck was having a nighttime confrontation with a nurse who insisted on putting him into uncomfortable positions. I actually had to bite my tongue to keep from entering the fray. He finally gave in, looking very pleased with himself, and stated as if giving royal permission, "Oh, go ahead. I'm putty in your hands." The two were a bonded couple after that.

- Try to figure out ways of dealing with the physical discomforts inherent in the hospital situation. In one hospital, Chuck and I were in a room that overlooked the Lifeflight helicopter pad. Fortunately, I'd brought along ear plugs and sleep masks for both of us.

- Offer distractions. During his chemotherapy, Chuck listened to Beethoven CDs with the best headphones we could afford. We played infinite games of gin and its variations.

- If you have a calming hobby yourself, see if it helps calm the patient. Having you sit there knitting, for instance, or tying flies, may be very homey and reassuring. On the other hand, it might drive the patient bonkers. Ask.

- If you and the patient have an erotic relationship, nurture it in the hospital setting as much as the patient's physical condition permits. Ask the physician what is and is not okay; don't be shy. Nothing is so empowering, non-invalid- and non-hospital-like as furtive hanky panky, especially with the danger of being walked in upon. Nearly every hospital room has a supply of KY jelly. Reread "that one chapter" in Hemingway's *A Farewell to Arms*.

Being a Good Citizen of the Hospital Ward

The more at home you are in the ward, the more safe and comfortable your patient will feel. To do so, become a good ward citizen. Here are my suggestions for making yourself a tolerated feature on a busy hospital ward.

- **Try not to betray an attitude that implies stereotypes.** Doctors, nurses, and staff members come in all sizes, ages, ethnicities, genders, and gender preferences. Don't assume that little blonde female is the head surgeon, and that tall distinguished gray-haired guy is the occupational therapist.

- **Be self-sufficient.** Never ask a staff member to be responsible for your own comfort as a sentinel. The ward, they are likely to remind you, is not a hotel. Bring your own water, snacks, hand-washies, pillow, blanket, book (see the Sentinel's Overnight Kit, in the next chapter). Don't snack from the food in the nurses' lounge. In fact, don't go into the lounge at all.

- **Help out, but ask first.** "I don't want to be in the way, but . . ." is a good way to start. Then, "If you show me what to do, I can empty the emesis (vomiting) basin or the bedpan." "I'll be glad to refill the water/ice pitcher." "If you help me figure it out, I'll be glad to help change [the patient's] hospital gown."

- **If you see an opportunity to commit ordinary kindness, take it.** Clear off the patient's meal tray and carry it to the waiting cart. If the charge nurse drops his pen while multitasking, pick it up and hand it over. With a smile. If you see litter on the floor, pick it up and throw it away. Then wash your hands.

- **Think before you invade privacy.** The whole staff is wearing pajama-like scrubs or loose uniforms, and the whole place is full of biology. So it might seem natural to ask almost anybody almost any personal question, or make any personal observation, or perform almost any little acts of personal intimacy. But that can be perceived as intrusive. Unless you already have established a relationship with a staff member, don't ask, "Do you have children?" "How did you get that scar?" "Do you think [the respiratory therapist, for instance] is gay?" "I'll bet you've had Botox." "I'll bet your feet really spread in those things." "Here, let me tuck that in for you." "Where does it itch? Here? Here?"

- **Be globally polite.** You'll be dealing with staff people from all over the world, many of them learning English as a second language. Rather than telling someone to "get somebody in here who speaks English!" say, "I'm having some trouble understanding you. Please slow down a little." If that doesn't work, repeat back what you think the person has said, in short easy sentences or by demonstrating. "You pull the bed rail up and anchor it like *this*?"

- **Respect the pressure on the nurses, including their time spent "charting."** Don't interrupt! No matter how long the shift, how many patients they were responsible for, and what crises have occurred, your nurses may not go home until everything is charted. This means filling in every blank, initialing every action, documenting every encounter in writing (or on the computer) demanded by bureaucracy.

HOSPITAL GOWNS

The purpose of the gown is to designate which ones are the patients. That's why almost all hospital gowns have that blue design, or are blue all over. And it is why you, the sentinel, should not wear one for sleep-wear or to protect your silk tie or for any other purpose.

If there is a crisis and you go for help in a gown, you will confuse everybody, and it will be difficult for you to act with confidence and authority. Whatever you do, when you wake up sweaty with your hair all sticking up at 11 P.M. and decide in a rage to search out the furnace room in the basement to ask them to turn down the heat in the patient's room, *do not* go down there wearing a hospital gown. Especially barefoot.

Many gowns will have missing or broken ties and snaps. The search for an intact gown of the right size and style (IV accessible, for instance) may prove fruitless. Note that one of the supplies in your Sentinel Kit is a packet of safety pins.

If a supply of gowns is readily available, try to keep an extra one on hand in case of spills, etc., and to carry along if the patient is transferred to another location.

Modesty

Most hospital gowns today are designed for modesty, but some are not. If your patient is permitted to get out of bed, make sure that everything is covered. You may need to tie one gown in back, and a second gown bathrobe-style, tied in front.

Many of the well-designed gowns accomplish tush coverage by closing at an angle or at the side. When you first encounter such a gown, it will seem as if the gown is malformed.

Sleeves

Some gowns have three sleeves. These are downright scary. Hint: one arm wears two sleeves, one over the other, to provide an extra panel in back for reliable tush coverage. The tie goes at the side.

Some have one sleeve. Or so it appears. In fact, the nonsleeve side is present but not sewn together at the shoulder. Instead, it has snaps along the top. This allows any IV tubing to exit freely, rather than be encumbered by a sleeve. Lay the robe out flat. Find the neck area (identified by a tab, or by border trim) and place it at the top. Find the one identifiable sleeve on either side of the neck line. Now follow the neck border in the *other direction* until it turns into snaps. Pinning it down firmly with one hand, explore until you come to a length of gown that also has snaps. Snap the snaps together and Voilà! You now have a gown with two sleeves.

When there is a snap sleeve, it is frequently combined with the third sleeve. Snap the sleeve first, and hold it up to determine which patient arm needs it for the IV. Then start with a real sleeve on the other, unencumbered arm; across the front to the snap sleeve, and then wind it around in back for the third sleeve on top of the original one. Try not to wind yourself into the gown.

ELEVEN

The Vigilant Sentinel

Night Duty and the Understaffed Ward

Having the sentinel stay overnight is safest and most reassuring for the patient, but hard on the sentinel and also on the staff. How would *you* feel if you were they? They worry that you will be watching their every move, and heaven forbid you catch them on a popcorn break. You will be bugging them every third minute about "I forgot my toothpaste, where can I get some?" And "It's too noisy in here to sleep, can't you talk softer?"

The overnight sentinel's goal is to maintain good ward citizenship while at the same time performing the sentinel's two duties of normalizing the environment and keeping the patient safe. Here are my suggestions:

- Think about the night while it's still daytime. Map out the ward. Where is the bathroom you can use? Where are the exit sign, the nearest stairs, and elevator? Where is the fire extinguisher and how does it work?

- Make sure that you have a flashlight so that you can see if you have to walk around or leave the room in the night.

- Figure out how you're going to sleep: where, and on what. Make sure that your sleeping arrangement doesn't impede free access to the patient.

- *The folding cot:* Figure it out *before* bedtime. It must be completely unfolded *and the legs braced.* Hospital cots come alive at around 10 P.M. If one of them takes against you, it can fold up in the middle of the night just like a PBJ sandwich on Wonder Bread, and you are the PBJ.

- *The reclining chair:* These all have a slippery shiny surface, and weigh as much as a baby hippo. If you yourself weigh less than 150 pounds, you will need assistance from a larger person to get it to recline. Make sure it reclines fully, or it too can fold up—not like Wonder Bread, but enough so that you wake in the night slithering down into a heap on the floor.

- *Two or three chairs pushed together:* This is obvious, but sometimes doesn't become so until the middle of the night: Make sure that they are wedged in position so a gap does not appear underneath your tush.

THE SENTINEL'S OVERNIGHT KIT

- Leave valuables at home. Ideally, carry your ID and cash in a money belt and wear it.

- Sleeping bag, if at all possible.

- Sleeping outfit for the sentinel. Sweats are good.

- Eye mask, one for you and one for patient, for blocking out bright lights carried by nurses.

- Really effective ear plugs: I recommend the MACK variety. Again, one set for you and one for patient.

- Flashlight for finding your way around a dim hospital room.

THE SENTINEL'S OVERNIGHT KIT *(continued)*

- Packet of safety pins for malfunctioning hospital gowns for patient.

- Prescriptions and any OTC medication you might need.

- Refillable water bottle. (Water source: fountain in hallway.)

- A source of hand sanitizing that doesn't require water. Wrapped individual washcloths or leave-on hand cleanser containing between 60 and 90 percent alcohol (Not less!).

- Cosmetics, toiletries including oral and hair care, including, ideally, face and body cleansers that are already moistened and don't require water.

- Small hand mirror if you really care how you look.

- Entertainment for you and patient: books, games, deck of cards, TV guide in case your hospital is on a different provider than your home.

- A piercing whistle, worn round your neck and tucked into your shirt, to be used only in the most rare and urgent crises.

THE UNDERSTAFFED WARD

We are in the midst of a severe shortage of nurses and hospital staff. You and the patient are likely to find yourselves in an understaffed ward.[18] Among the missing are RNs and LPNs.

---

18. In an article published in the September/October 2005 issue of *Nursing Economics*, Dr. Peter Buerhaus and associates found that the majority of RNs (79 percent) and Chief Nursing Officers (68 percent) believe the nursing shortage is affecting the overall quality of patient care in hospitals and other settings, including long-term care facilities, ambulatory care settings, and student health centers. Most hospital RNs (93 percent) report major problems with having enough time to maintain patient safety, detect complications early, and collaborate with other team members.

Registered nurses are college-educated nursing school graduates. RNs monitor the monitors and respond to alarms, administer injections and intravenous medications, operate technical equipment such as ventilators and intravenous pumps, alert physicians when there is a crisis, and protect patients from doctors' inexperience, doctors from loss of face, and everybody from loss of faith. With higher patient loads, longer shifts, and greatly increased technical responsibilities, they're lucky if they have time and energy for just the basics.

Licensed practical nurses are the nurses who take vital signs (blood pressure, pulse, weight), change sterile dressings, give oral medications, prepare patients for surgery, and provide comfort care—bathing, treating bed sores, making sure the right meals are served to the right patient.

Non-medically trained staff members are also in short supply. This means that fresh laundry, bed changing, and food delivery may be delayed; that ordinary supplies can run out without being reordered; that the person who pushes the patient's wheelchair may not have a clear idea of the risks involved, much less the best route to the destination.

Is Your Ward Understaffed?

To find out, just observe. What is the atmosphere on the ward? Do the nurses look frazzled? Do they power-walk from patient to patient? Do they multitask, writing notes while they fill syringes while they answer the phone while they push along a wheelchair with one foot? Is there hardly any small talk going on, just orders and responses? Do they sigh a lot? Seem never to sit down? How much ground do you think each of them covers in a day—and what percentage of their shift time is spent just power-walking from patient to desk to patient?

At the change of each shift, does your new nurse have complete and accurate information on you? Do you have to remind your nurse for medication doses or about diet restrictions?

Another key observation: Who's filling the comfort jobs of changing sheets, serving and clearing meals, cleaning the floors? Is English the first language for *any* of them? Do they look tired and move as if in pain? For many, this is likely to be a second or third job.

Finally, during times of transition and stress, even a well-staffed ward can be relatively short-handed. Moving into new hospital space or installing a new computer system can be very disruptive. A tragedy on the ward, or one that affects a key member of the staff, can affect everybody's mood and efficiency.

What Can You Do?

To be an effective sentinel in an understaffed or stressed ward, you must step in and help just as much as you feel able.

If you can document just how stressed the staff is, consider filing a complaint *on behalf of the staff.* Even if it may appear that only one or two staff members are not up to snuff, it is much more likely that the problem is basically due to understaffing and poor morale.

Call the Joint Commission on Accreditation of Healthcare Organization's complaint line, 800-994-6610 (Weekdays, 8:30 A.M. to 5 P.M. Central Time). Or write the problem in a short form and e-mail it to www.complaints@jcaho.org, or download a form at www.jcaho.org (click on "General Public" and then on "Go to report a complaint"). This will only be effective if your hospital is a JCAHO accredited facility.

Don't think of yourself as a tattletale, but as a whistleblower on the side of the staff.

TWELVE

The Hypervigilant Sentinel

We turn now from vigilance to hypervigilance. Hypervigilance means that you are always on the alert for something to go wrong, and always thinking ahead what to do if something does. You may have to step in and do things far beyond what you expected.

There are two situations that are particularly likely to be triggers for hypervigilance: physician unresponsiveness and a very sick patient in an understaffed ward.

PHYSICIAN UNRESPONSIVENESS

By this I mean that a crisis is occurring but the physician is, well, unresponsive. The reason doesn't matter, nor does the nature of the crisis itself. When this happens, you may need to go to the nurses and do whatever you need to have them get appropriate help. Fortunately, your very presence as sentinel has increased the chances of your success in this regard.

First, it is infinitely comforting for the patient just to know you are right there, an intimate connection to normal health and life. A patient who feels loved and watched is spared the kind of anxiety that can precipitate a crisis all by itself.

Second, you have very likely earned the good opinion of the staff on your ward, a reputation for being a good citizen who is there to help them, not harass them. So you, too, can be spared anxiety. You know that if you really need help, they'll be there for you.

Third, you are extra insurance that if a crisis occurs, it will be recognized and dealt with promptly. That's because you are yourself an exquisitely sensitive monitor of the patient's condition.

The Human Monitor

Sure, there are monitors attached to your patient. But each monitor is programmed with a preset "normal range." The monitor will not alarm until the out-of-range point is reached. However, it's rare for a disaster to occur from one heartbeat to the next; the human body is very sturdy, and fights off most disasters with vigor. So there's a period of time between when the first signs of trouble occur and when the monitor goes off.

If a nurse could watch each and every monitor and each and every patient all the time, chances are such trouble triggers would be picked up nearly immediately, because the nurse would see a trend in the tracking of at least one monitor—would see the trend, that is, before it actually reached the out-of-range mark.

But that really defeats the whole labor-saving point of the monitors. Besides, there are three important "vital signs" the monitor can't measure: how the patient is feeling, how he is behaving, and what the *trend* is in vital signs on the monitors. It used to be that nurses tracked this, but these days you, and they, cannot count on the staffing to do so.

But you, the sentinel, can be crucial in this effort.

What can the patient tell you?

A self-aware and alert patient often knows that something is going wrong before a doctor or a monitor can find it.

Once in the middle of the night, Chuck said to me "I've got another air pocket in my lung; it's hard to breathe." By this time, he'd had five air pockets treated by tubes, so he knew what he was talking about. I told the nurses, who listened to his chest and then looked at the monitors. Everything looked okay.

How is the patient behaving? Is he changing for the worse?

When you've sat as a sentinel for a few hours, you get a sense of your patient's "normal" state. That's the state of alertness, coherence, and comfort that is usual for him or her at this time with this condition.

Over the next hour, Chuck got worse. I asked the nurse to page the Fellow in lung surgery. The Fellow ordered a chest X ray, and read it as showing no air pocket, and stomped out furious at having been called at home.

As Chuck had more and more trouble breathing, he stopped talking to me except in short phrases. He kept trying to find a better position in which to breathe. I held his hand, and asked the nurses to start him on oxygen. They did so; they were worried too, but afraid to page the Fellow again; he'd yelled at all of us so effectively the first time.

Do the monitor readings show an ominous trend, even if the readings are still within "normal" range and the alarm isn't going off?

Every patient has his own range of normal, which may be very different from normal for a healthy person. We should probably call it an "expected" range, given the nature of illness and condition of the patient, rather than a normal range.

If you have been sitting there for hours, you probably have an idea of your own patient's expected range on each of the usual monitors: heart rate, blood pressure, and pulse oximeter, which measures how well-saturated the blood is with oxygen.

Of course the readings will bounce around, depending on the patient's activity. It's the trend over time that matters. Remember, the monitor will not alarm until the numbers go outside a preset "expected" range.

During the hours that Chuck was sure he had an air pocket in his lung, the monitors stayed in the expected range. Well, yes; but his "pulse ox" dropped from an "expected" 97 percent to an "expected" 93 percent; his blood pressure dropped down from an "expected" 120/80 to an "expected" 95/65, and his heart rate rose to the top of his "expected" range, from 68 to 110.

Finally, at about 4 A.M., I stalked into the nurses' station and started talking firmly and then yelling. Instead of calling security, the blessed souls paged the senior surgeon and handed me the phone. I yelled at him, too, and he came running in; took one look and listen, then ran for the chest tube tray. By this time Chuck was grey and incoherent. There was no time for general anesthesia or even for novacaine; I was Chuck's anesthesia, holding him tightly still and talking to him until with enormous effort the surgeon inserted the life-saving tube and the trapped air in the chest came out with a whoosh.

We were all sweaty and trembling, but Chuck was breathing normally.

CRISIS TRIGGERS

- The patient is less than twenty-four hours out of major surgery.

- There has been a major change in condition within the last twenty-four hours.

- The patient has had a change in the amount of oxygen being given, either increased or decreased.

- The patient is on a new pain medication, has had an increase or decrease in pain medicine, or has had a change from oral pain medication to medication given by injection (in a muscle, vein, or spinal fluid.)

A VERY SICK PATIENT IN AN UNDERSTAFFED WARD

The critical nursing shortage in America puts patients at risk. As Sentinel, you may find it necessary to step in to help in ways you never dreamed of. At one point, Chuck had a procedure in which a kind of "glue" was injected through one of his chest tubes. The "glue" was supposed to coat the entire lining of his chest cavity, so that the air pocket itself would stick to the lining, healing itself and allowing the removal of the suction tube. For that to happen, he needed to be rotated slowly and constantly in all directions. He couldn't turn on his own; he was impeded by all the tubes.

I was given the task of standing at the foot of the bed, pressing the bed buttons to raise and lower his chest, then climbing up on the bed to help him turn from side to side without damage to the tubes. It was painful for him—for us both. The process went on for over an hour. The nurses were so relieved not to have to take so much time with only one patient.

In the book *Truth & Beauty, a Memoir of a Friendship,* by novelist Ann Patchett (HarperCollins 2004, pp. 189–191), Patchett gives a harrowing example of being put to the test. Her friend Lucy had just had drastic surgery on her jaw, plus the removal of a bone in her lower leg to use as a jaw graft.

When Patchett arrived at NYU Medical Center hours after the surgery, she found Lucy conscious but in grave danger: vomiting frequently, but bandaged and restrained in such a way that she couldn't raise or turn her head. Fortunately, another friend had been present and stood by with a suction tube, preventing Lucy from choking on the vomit.

There were two nurses on the floor. They were too busy to even look in on Lucy. The two friends suctioned her, bathed her, and changed the sheets. In the following days, when the nurses were too overwhelmed to give Lucy her intravenous pain medication on time, Patchett would track them down and remind them, *"repeatedly, firmly, and, when it was absolutely necessary, unkindly."* She found clean sheets and towels and without asking permission (and with no one stopping her), took over the task of being Lucy's personal RN, LPN, and housekeeper.

As she said, the nurses were grateful because, as in Chuck's case, it gave them "one less patient to worry about."

If you find yourself in this kind of situation, my advice is that you do what you know needs to be done. Do not waste time berating the staff. If you don't know how something works, such as suction or oxygen, demand ("repeatedly, firmly, and, when absolutely necessary, unkindly") that you be shown, and then if you need to, you can do it yourself.

There is nothing I know of to protect an individual patient and Sentinel from being placed in this position. If you're rich, you can hire a private nurse, if you can find one, but that nurse may not be a solution. Many patients report that the private nurse didn't know how to handle the equipment, nor its location, and was not comfortable communicating with the ward nurses. The private nurse didn't know the physicians in charge of the patient, and didn't know whom to call. Sometimes, the private nurse was asked—firmly—to leave her patient and go and help the overworked nurses on the ward.

This can happen no matter how rich, famous, respected, or well connected the patient or the Sentinel might be. Does it help to be a health care CEO, CFO, or member of the Board of Directors? I can't imagine how. I wonder what they would say about it. Maybe I'll hear from one of them; I'll let you know if I do.

THIRTEEN

The Sentinel in Transit

When Chuck was at MD Anderson and UCSD for the air pockets, he needed to travel down to the basement for a chest X ray almost every day for the total eight weeks. That's not unusual; patients often need studies or treatments performed in other parts of the hospital: an MRI in radiology, an echocardiogram stress test in cardiology, a trip back to the operating room to fix a minor problem, and so on.

Traveling within the hospital can be tiring for everybody. Once in awhile, it can be dangerous: the patient takes a turn for the worse when there's no staff person around who knows what to do; or equipment malfunctions—there is a problem with the IV, the oxygen, or the urine catheter; or there's a traffic accident with the means of transport: the wheelchair or the gurney (a stretcher on wheels) collides with something, breaks down, or somehow ejects the patient.

As sentinel, you may be able to make transit a lot safer.

PREVENTION

Understand the nature of the excursion: Ask your nurse. Popping down to radiology for a routine X ray is one thing. An invasive procedure, involving even minor pain or nausea, is another. A patient who's never had a CT scan needs to be told ahead of time about the need to be in a tunnel machine, or one that rotates around him. If he's never had an MRI, he needs to know it too is a tunnel experience and also be prepared for the erratic banging (Chuck said it reminded him of our Sara as a teen, in the early phase of her drum lessons.)

- If it looks as though your trip may interfere with the timing of a medication dose, especially for pain, flag this to the nurse.

- Read the section at the end of this chapter on MRI safety.

- Is the patient going to miss a meal or a therapy treatment because of the trip? Ask the nurse what to do.

- Is there likely to be anything you could take along that would add to the patient's comfort? It gets mighty cold down in the radiology suite. Sometimes they keep warm blankets down there. Sometimes they run out.

Check on the Patient

- If the patient is alert and competent, ask him if he feels up to the coming trip.

- If your instinct tells you that the patient is getting ready to get sicker, tell the nurse before you leave the ward. Ask how stressful the trip and test are likely to be. If you run into trouble on the way, what should you do? Can the test be safely postponed?

Check on the Equipment

As soon as you know a transit is scheduled within the next hour, check the tubes, fluids, oxygen, and medication. The nurse will do this too, if there is time. If the ward is overstaffed, don't count on it.

- When the urine bag becomes two-thirds full, ask that it be emptied before the journey.

- When the IV looks as if there is less than half in the bottle, ask the nurse this: "Could the IV be slowed down if it looks as if it's going to run dry while we're en route? Or would that be dangerous? Should we start with a full container?" This will focus his mind and relieve yours.

Check on the Oxygen Supply

Learn as much as you can about the oxygen situation. For a patient in bed, the oxygen supply comes from the wall outlet, and you don't have to worry about running out. A gauge on the wall regulates flow—that is how much oxygen flows into the patient's mask or tubing every minute. Ask the nurse how many "liters per minute" the patient is getting. (Don't worry about the "liters" part; metrics has nothing to do with it.) You just want to know the normal amount your patient needs, in case the gauge has to be re-set during transit.

When the patient is in transit, the oxygen must come from a tube connected to a portable oxygen tank. This tank is filled with oxygen under high pressure so a lot of it can fit in the tank. The tank goes along with the patient—either hung on the gurney or wheelchair, or in a little wheeled basket of its own.

There are two possible problems with this arrangement:

1. The tank may run out of oxygen. For this reason, make sure you are leaving with a reasonably full tank. Ask your nurse to double check. If you're told, "Oh don't worry, they'll have full ones at [your destination]" don't buy it. They may have full tanks, but there may not be anyone free to install one. Those things are really heavy and need a special wrench to turn them on. Insist on a full one.

Ask the nurse or respiratory therapist to show you how to tell whether the tank is running low. It's easy, there's a gauge with the caution area usually in yellow and the "nearly empty" in red. But every make of tank is a little different.

2. The tubing may accidentally get yanked out of the attachment to the tank. When this happens, it pops off like a champagne cork (because the oxygen is pressurized) and the oxygen coming out of the tank continues to flow. In order to reattach the tubing to the tank, you must turn the tank off, reattach the tubing to the nozzle, turn the tank on again, and adjust the flow. Try to get someone to show you how to do this before leaving the ward. It isn't hard, and you'll feel more in control knowing.

Be Prepared Yourself

On anything other than a short, routine trip, I learned, it's a good idea to take along a vomiting basin; a pair of gloves for yourself; an extra hospital gown (with intact ties) for the patient; and a deck of cards either for you and the patient to play or for you waiting for the patient to play solitaire.

TRANSPORTATION

Usually, the patient is not allowed to walk to where he's going, even if he has been walking comfortably for days around the ward.

It is rare for a licensed or registered nurse to accompany the trip. The person who pushes the wheelchair or gurney almost never has had medical training and may be someone with whom you do not share fluency in a common language.

Getting Around with Your Patient

You may have an attendant who is very adept at transporting patients, or you may get a beginner. In either event, you need to know what transporting a patient entails, and what to do to prevent or deal with a glitch.

The Gurney

It is a padded stretcher on wheels. Alert patients may dislike the gurney because it is unpleasant to travel on one's back, not being able to see ahead and anticipate what's coming up. But it may be the best way to travel if the patient is attached to lots of equipment. An IV pole is attached to the gurney itself, and there is usually a stable shelf or other arrangement for oxygen canisters.

If you have to deal with the gurney yourself:

- Make sure the gurney is "anchored" so it won't move when the patient is transferred, or transfers him/herself, on and off. There is a brake near one of the wheels. Find it and use it, if your attendant forgets.

- Make sure the side rails are up for the ride, even if the patient is alert, sane, and really, really annoyed at the idea.

- Make sure the patient is strapped in, again over any objections. Gurney accidents often occur when two gurneys collide whisking around a corner, and the rails may not prevent a patient from falling out.

- Make sure all tubing is securely inside the rails before you set off. Nothing more dangerous or humiliating than finding yourself lassoed by the IV.

- If it is safe, and the patient is alert, elevate the head so he can see where he's headed.

The Wheelchair

The hospital model of the wheelchair bears some resemblance to a grocery cart: it must be pushed, many people have used it to transport loads of varying weights, and one of the wheels may be out of alignment. Accidents with wheelchairs occur when the patient trips on getting in or out, falls out, or tips backwards. This can happen on rough, bumpy, or steep terrain, when the equipment is faulty, and when the correct procedures are not followed.

- Check it out as you see the attendant wheeling it in. Does it seem to fight and reassert itself in a wrong direction? Ask the attendant, pointing and acting out if you don't speak a mutual language. If the diagnosis is correct, appeal to the least busy nurse you can find to get a better wheelchair.

- Before your patient gets in or out of the chair, make sure of three things:

  1. The chair is braked—anchored so it can't wiggle around.

  2. The footrests are up and out of the way.

  3. You have a plan to help your patient out of the bed, down to the floor, and into the chair. If she has been in bed for a long time, sitting or standing up can produce momentary dizziness. Take it slowly.

- Once your patient is in the chair, lower the footrests and make sure s/he is comfortable. Need a pillow? Take it off the bed. Need a blanket? Ask for one.

- Strap the patient in securely.

- Make sure any attachable equipment is properly attached. Make sure the IV pole is settled into the built-in IV pole holder so that it doesn't tend to collapse itself at the first bump. Make sure the urine bag is hooked on to the chair and is lower than the patient's bottom (It works by gravity.)

- The oxygen tank or suction pump may have to travel alongside on little wheeled baskets of their own. If the attendant allows it, take over pushing the wheeled basket yourself so that the attendant can be fully devoted to the wheelchair.

- Remember to reverse all these procedures when the patient gets out at your destination, and perform them all over again when he gets back in, and reverse them again when you're back on the ward, and on and on ad infinitum.

Trouble in Transit

The patient feels bad and looks worrisome

He is pale or flushed, sweaty, working to breathe.

If oxygen is available, place the mask on the patient and turn the flow on so that the needle points at the number 3 (it is flowing at 3 liters per minute.) If the oxygen is already flowing, turn it up by two liters/minute.

At the same time, yell for the nearest white coat. If you can't find a medically trained person in the vicinity, and the patient is not getting better, blow your whistle.

The urine bag becomes filled to capacity

Urine drains into the urine bag from tubing that enters the bladder. If the bag fills up, the only place for newly-produced urine to go is into the ever more bulging bladder.

It's not a life-threatening emergency, but it can feel like one to the patient. What to do? Stop along the way at any white coat, and ask for help. It should take less than a minute to deal with the problem.

Only if you can't find help, resort to the following strategy: Observe the bag. There is a clamp that, when released, will allow the urine to drain. Ask the attendant to help you hold the vomit basin you brought along, for the urine to drain into. Put on your gloves and open the drain. (If you forgot gloves, don't worry; urine is a pretty sterile bodily fluid.)

Drain enough to relieve the pressure in the bladder; the patient will say "when." Empty the urine-filled basin into a toilet if you pass a restroom. If you don't see a restroom near, leave the basin on a surface (windowsill, etc.) with a towel over it and, if you have a pencil and paper, a sign that says "Full of pee! Sorry!"

The IV looks as if it is going to run dry while you're in transit

If the nurse said that it probably wouldn't run dry, and that if it did, it wouldn't be a problem, just try to slow down the rate that the drops are falling. Do not try to do this on your own; find any white coat and ask him or her to slow down the flow.

If the nurse led you to believe that the IV would not, should not, must not run dry, get yourself to a medical person and explain the situation; ask him to call the patient's ward and get instructions.

Your patient requires a constant source of oxygen

The higher the flow your patient needs, the faster the tank will empty.

Keep your eye on the tank's fullness gauge. If the needle is hovering close to the red zone, start seeking out sources of oxygen tanks, wherever you are. Stop any white coat, or indeed any useful-looking employee. Don't wait until the needle hits red. It takes time to locate and change a tank.

THE MRI SUITE

This is perhaps the most potentially dangerous destination in the hospital.

An MRI is powered by a magnet stronger than any you can imagine. It is so strong that it lines up subatomic particles in the body! This means that any substance capable of being magnetized will come under its spell.

Magnetizable objects of any size will "home into" the magnet at top speed, regardless of what's in the way, including your head. Such objects have included "oxygen cylinders, IV poles, parts of a forklift, a helium cylinder, a mop bucket, a laundry cart, a chair, a ladder, a patient lift, a light fixture, a floor buffer, a pulse oximeter, a transformer, tools, scissors, and traction weights [weights used for keeping a leg elevated on pulleys.]"[19]

Any device implanted within the patient's body must be checked for MRI safety. The following are especially dangerous: cochlear implants, internal or external cardiac pacemakers, implantable infusion pumps, and cerebral aneurysm clips. "Devices that contain a magnet that might move or become demagnetized, such as dental implants or prostheses with magnetic components may also be adversely affected by the MRI."[20]

If anyone in the MRI room has any metallic fragment (shrapnel, bullets) or implants within their body, the magnet will make the metal get hot and move around. The tiniest metal fragment embedded in an eye could move around and cause blindness. Even metallic eye makeup will react, making the eyelids flutter, and a tattoo will become inflamed and itch. Loose jewelry will be pulled off limbs (and possibly out of the belly button) to the mother magnet.

There are no federal regulations for MRI safety, whether the MRI is located in hospital or in a shopping mall. Be careful!

---

19. "Patient Death Illustrates the Importance of Adhering to Safety Precautions in Magnetic Resonance Environments" *ECRI*, August 6, 2001.
20. Ibid.

PART THREE

Afterwards

FOURTEEN

Aftermath

January 4, 2002–June 5, 2003

At last, by June of 2002, Chuck was free of chest tubes and really started to recuperate, taking walks on the beach, enjoying real meals. We started seeing our friends, and resumed a good part of our normal life. (Except the dancing. For some reason, Chuck just didn't have the stamina, he said, not making eye contact, for the cha cha. I shall always wonder about that.)

Then came time for the radiation part of the protocol. This was to prevent recurrences from microscopic tumors that might have survived chemo and surgery. The radiation was not as debilitating as we had feared. As a routine, Chuck was put on the anti-inflammatory steroid Prednisone, to try to prevent scarring of the esophagus, airways, lung tissue, and blood vessels in the chest.

By September, despite the tumor's destruction of the crucial nerve that triggers the right diaphragm, the surgical loss of a third of his lung tissue on the right, and the effects of radiation, Chuck felt really good. Then in October, he started "consolidation chemotherapy," the final stage of the MD Anderson protocol.

But this time the chemotherapy was fraught with minor problems and seemed to be more debilitating. Finally, Chuck chose to opt out of the rest of the treatment, in December 2002. But he didn't bounce back.

The scar-preventive Prednisone was being decreased. And we both worried that scarring was occurring. Over the winter and spring, he grew increasingly fatigued, developed a cough, and had trouble talking.

For the first time, in the spring, he experienced some real pain. By the end of May 2003, he had had every test known to man or woman, had seen every expert anyone could suggest, and no cause or solution could be found. A high-resolution CT performed May 30 showed "no residual or new tumor."

On June 5, 2003, I awoke at dawn to find him sharing my pillow, breathing the heavy Kussmaul sighs of impending death, hemorrhaging from his mouth. He had such a calm, pleased look on his face, but he was cold and there was so much blood. And I couldn't find a pulse.

I wanted just to hold him, but all my training forced me to try to give him CPR. I couldn't even get him into a position for resuscitation to be effective. By the time the paramedics arrived, Chuck was dead. I think he had lost his entire blood volume in less than ten minutes.

The first person I called was my senior partner, Fred Frumin. I could count on him to take over calmly, without shock or undue distress at the scene. He stayed with me as the day progressed, through the terrible calls to Sara and to Chuck's father; through the hasty cemetery arrangements, through a frustrating encounter with the Eye Bank; through the transfer of Chuck's body to the funeral home; through the removal of the mattress and the cutting of a big person-shaped hole in the carpet, saturated with blood.

He stayed with me until Sara arrived at 5 that afternoon.

I knew I should have permitted an autopsy. I didn't. The "fine-tuned" CT of the week before had shown no evidence of remaining or new cancer. Our doctors told me that unavoidable, unpredictable radiation damage probably had eroded large blood vessels in the chest. They said that the rare patients who are in the hospital when this occurs, and who survive it, report it as a painless event.

FIFTEEN

Coping and Questioning

Sara stayed with me for nearly three months, thanks to the kindness of the federal judge for whom she was clerking. She tells me I cried all the time, and I believe her.

She did everything from choosing the casket and arranging the funeral to standing up at the packed memorial service and saying thank you, from taking care of her devastated Grandpa Ben to making me eat, from cowriting Chuck's epitaph to teaching me how to find my way to the cemetery.

She also had to deal with the household problems. By law, the bed mattress and the bedroom carpet had to be taken out because they were saturated with blood and thus hazardous waste. But the carpet was continuous throughout the house, and so all of it was taken out and replaced. We rented a bed for me for weeks, until we felt able to go shop for a new mattress.

Finally I told her I could manage okay with our circle of friends, and that she should get back to work.

A few weeks after Sara went back to Baltimore, I started work myself, a few hours a day. I looked so terrible that sometimes I would walk into an exam room to see a family I'd known for years, and the baby would start to cry and the mother would start to cry and the young children would hide behind her. Gradually I got better, with a lot of help and time.

I visited Chuck's grave every day early before going to work. I left fresh flowers, and every night the deer came and ate them. Finally, I got some deer repellent spray and sprayed the flowers, which worked, but I accidentally left the spray bottle open in the trunk of the car. I tried car washes, scrubbing, and finally something called "Anti-Icky-Poo," which worked, sort of. Nobody is likely to steal my Prius, though.

During the last weeks of 2003, I became increasingly frantic. I couldn't seem to get control of anything. Winter rains flooded the house, rats ate the air ducts, an invasion of termites arrived right under my computer station. A parade of experts arrived nearly weekly: the house painters, the flood guys, drywall guys, exterminators of rats and then of termites, and plumbers galore. When I showed up in February for my very first solo appointment with our tax accountant of twenty years, I was told by the secretary that I had been transferred to "the new guy." The new guy barely knew my name, never said a word about Chuck's death, and told me that I needed to pay the IRS $32,000 by April 15.

Happily, family and friends stepped in. I felt like a balloon in a game where all the players were determined to keep it safely airborne, sometimes reaching way far out to keep it from hurtling downward or into a sharp object.

By March 2004, I started finally to see colors in the world again. The first time I remember laughing was when one of the guys, a very large one, was ascending the ladder into the attic in search of more rats in the air ducts. He was telling me a story about a herd of elk that got drunk on rotten apples in a small town. Halfway into the hole, the guy started imitating how the elk wove and staggered down the streets of the town, and started laughing, and he got stuck. The more he laughed, the more he stuck, and the more he laughed and stuck, the more I laughed.

When the rains finally stopped, Jack (my cosentinel at UCSD) and I returned to the Sunday ritual of running in Torrey Pines. On a specific trail bench overlooking the Pacific, you will find (if you look for it) a plaque that says "Chuck Nathanson: 1941–2003. He loved these trails." It is on the back of the bench, because plaques are not allowed. So it is a secret.

By January of 2004, I was able to return, tentatively, to thinking about what had happened. My main concern was that there might be a system error—a flaw in the way the local clinic was operating. It seemed possible to me that the "culture" of the practice of medicine there had broken down, leaving individual physicians unclear about each one's accountability. What other factor could explain the oversights of eight different physicians, in seven different departments?

My first act was to issue formal complaints about each of the involved physicians (excluding doctors-in-training) to the California Board of Medicine, for all the MDs, and to the California Board of Osteopathic Medicine, for the DO radiologist. My letters were detailed and, of course, were supported by the original documents.

Missed Diagnosis of Tumor on Chest X ray, January 31, 2000

- Emergency room physician for not following up on chest X ray he had ordered

- Radiologist for incomplete and ambiguous reading of chest X ray

- Admitting cardiologist for ignoring the student doctor's "fuzzy logic" interpretation of chest X ray, and for not even attempting to exclude the diagnosis of malignancy

- Discharging cardiologist (who also performed the outpatient follow-up) for never once mentioning the chest X ray in any report; and for taking on a diagnostic problem outside his realm of competence as lipid specialist

- Internist, who recognized that the diagnosis of an "idiopathic" condition was inadequate, but who made no coherent plan to address this or to follow-up with the specialist

Misdiagnosis of Tumor as Cancer of Unknown Primary Site, November 2001

- Pulmonologist, who did not include the possibility of malignant thymoma in her biopsy request, despite the fact that the radiologist had suggested it as a major possibility

- Pathologist, for failing to state whether the biopsy sample was adequate, and for failing to look for thymoma in the samples of the tumor from the anterior mediastinum. (Thymoma is the *most common cause* of a mass in the anterior mediastinum.)

- Hematologist for taking on the role of oncologist without disclosing his credentials; for giving as a definitive diagnosis one that was really a diagnosis of exclusion; for not excluding the most likely tumor type (thymoma); for giving the diagnosis of a rapidly fatal, untreatable tumor in a rushed and impersonal manner, with no follow-up appointment; and for refusing to honor a request for a second opinion.

RESULTS

The State (appointed by the Governor) Medical Board Quality Control Committee sent me form letters exonerating each of the medical doctors.

The Osteopathic Board initially found that the radiologist was guilty of simple negligence.

STATE AND CONSUMER SERVICES AGENC\ GRAY DAVIS, Gover

OSTEOPATHIC MEDICAL BOARD OF CALIFORNIA
2720 GATEWAY OAKS DRIVE, SUITE 350
SACRAMENTO, CA 95833-4304
TELEPHONE: (916) 263-3100
FAX: (916) 263-3117

State of
California
Department of
Consumer
Affairs

⑤

June 24, 2003

Laura Nathanson, M.D., FAAP
▮▮▮▮ Caminito Pt. Del Mar
Del Mar, CA 92014

*Rescinded
and replaced
on July 10, 2003*

Re: ▮▮▮▮▮▮▮▮▮▮
     Our Ref No. 00 2002 1154

Dear Dr. Nathanson:

The Special Consultant has completed his evaluation of the x-ray of Mr. Charles Nathanson and supporting medical records.

At this time, the matter is closed with simple negligence. The Consultant came to this conclusion because Dr. ▮▮▮▮ interpretation of the radiograph is accurate though understating the pleural mass appearance. Dr. ▮▮▮▮ could have suggested appropriate follow-up studies such as a CT of the chest for further evaluation. This would comply with the standards of chest radiograph interpretation from the American College Radiology.

As the case has been completely reevaluated and the Consultant did not recommend any further action, the matter is closed without further action.

If you have any questions, please feel free to contact me.

Sincerely,

LINDA J. BERGMANN
EXECUTIVE DIRECTOR

LJB:ab

But this letter was followed by a retraction.

STATE AND CONSUMER SERVICES AGENCY   GRAY DAVIS, Gor

OSTEOPATHIC MEDICAL BOARD OF CALIFORNIA

State of California Department of
Consumer Affairs

2720 GATEWAY OAKS DRIVE, SUITE 350
SACRAMENTO, CA 95833-4304
TELEPHONE: (916) 263-3100
FAX: (916) 263-3117

July 10, 2003

Laura Nathanson, M.D., FAAP
███ Caminito Pt. Del Mar
Del Mar, CA 92014

Re: ████████████
       Our Ref No. 00 2002 1154

Dear Dr. Nathanson:

The letter we sent to you dated June 24, 2003 (Exhibit B) regarding the decision of your complaint is herewith rescinded as Dr. ███ explained the MAFI Code System ██████ ███ as follows:

> MAFI System is used for chest x-rays and mammography. A Code "0" means no further imaging is necessary. A Code "1" means that further investigation is necessary (reference Exhibit A). The patient with a Code 1 is placed on a computer list to the ordering physician. They or the MAFI coordinator have to acknowledge each patient with a Code 1 to do more imaging, biopsy, consultation or whatever is clinically necessary.

> Dr. ███ is not required to state what further imaging procedure is necessary, but he did notify the clinician that there was an abnormality and further work was necessary. The clinician then contacts the patient for further testing, etc.

For this reason, the case is considered closed.

If you have any questions, please feel free to contact me.

Sincerely,

Linda J. Bergmann
LINDA J. BERGMANN
EXECUTIVE DIRECTOR

LJB:ab

Enclosures

cc: ████████████

I stared at the retraction for quite awhile. For one thing, I couldn't understand how the executive director, with no medical credentials, could simply overturn the finding of negligence made by medical experts, based only on the word of the accused physician.

But I was much more concerned about the mysterious system referred to as "MAFI." (I never could find out what the letters stand for.) It appeared to me that under this system a radiologist was not required to read a film but merely to screen it as normal (Code 0) or abnormal (Code 1). It appeared to me that under MAFI, the responsibility for actually reading the film—deciding which aspects were abnormal, and why—had been transferred from the radiologist to the clinician. And from the letter, this system was being used both for all chest X rays and all mammograms!

I had never heard of such a thing.

WHAT I DID

I contacted the American College of Radiology, where a spokesperson told me that the ACR guidelines were just that, guidelines, and not enforceable.

I wrote to JCAHO, the Joint Commission on Accreditation of Health-care Organizations, including a copy of the osteopathic correspondence. I received in return a form letter stating that they were unable to investigate any incident occurring more than a year prior to the complaint.

I also considered a lawsuit. My attorney reminded me that it would be hard, as with any cancer case—but especially a rare cancer—to prove that any errors made a real difference in outcome. That is, one has to prove both liability and *causality*. Moreover, California has a $250,000 cap on "pain and suffering" awards. It would be very difficult to find someone who would take such an uncertain case on contingency.

Finally, she reminded me, the MD Anderson and Vanderbilt doctors should not have to spend their precious time flying around the country, testifying in court as expert witnesses.

Very kindly, she did have one of her staff research the question: Does the executive director of the Board of Osteopathy have the right to rescind a disciplinary decision of a medical expert, simply on the word of the accused doctor himself?

Here is the answer:

MEMORANDUM

TO: ▮▮▮▮▮▮▮▮

FROM: ▮▮▮▮▮▮

RE: Osteopathic Medical Board of California Executive Director Powers

DATE: November 12, 2003

<u>Question Presented</u>

Does the Executive Director Possess the Power to Reverse a Finding of Negligence Following an Ex Parte Communication?

<u>Short Answer</u>

Yes.

Section 1603 of the rules governing the Osteopathic Medical Board of California (attached) confers upon the executive director "all functions necessary to the proper dispatch of the business of the Board in connection with all investigative and administrative proceedings" except for those reserved to the "agency itself" under the Administrative Procedure Act, Section 11500. As the Administrative Procedure Act does not mention the agency's ability to overturn findings of negligence, that power is reserved to the executive director under Section 1603.

SIXTEEN

An Exercise in Futility

I couldn't just let it go.

From my first discoveries in Chuck's medical record, I had suspected a "system error." I couldn't help thinking that this MAFI code was a good candidate. As described by the radiologist, the MAFI code system removed accountability from the radiologists. The system appeared to expect that clinical physicians, untrained in reading chest X rays and mammograms, would suddenly be able to take over—and would be held solely accountable if they couldn't handle the task.

Of course, there was always the possibility that the radiologist was merely inventing an institutional excuse for an individual failing.

There was also the possibility that MAFI was truly in effect—if not in a written decree, then in the accepted behavior of physicians.

I needed to find out what exactly was going on in the radiology department.

When all my efforts at enlisting the support of professional/governmental agencies failed, I decided to consider publicity. This was in January 2004. Our local channel, KGTV, has an excellent reputation for responsible investigative reporting. With my attorney sitting in, I taped a fifteen-minute segment about the MAFI mystery, displaying Chuck's original X ray, the disastrous report by the radiologist, the initial finding of negligence by the Osteopathic Board, and the radiologist's self-exoneration using the MAFI system. I explained my concerns as clearly as I could.

KGTV would air the tape only if someone of professional standing would present the Institution's side of the story, or at least give an "unbiased" comment. I called several physicians of standing and experience, but no one (except for my partners) agreed to help. Finally, I wrote to a member of the Institution's board of directors who had been a friend of Chuck's and a member of his group, the San Diego Dialogue. I told him the whole story.

He couldn't find anyone to go on TV. However, greatly to his credit, he managed to set up a meeting for me with himself and four or five of the head honchos of the Institution.

I felt, accurately, that I would need moral support plus a witness at this meeting, but that the presence of an attorney—even my Sara—would be a dampener. My senior partner Fred Frumin was my first choice, and he graciously agreed to come with me.

I was impressed with the credentials of those gathered, and I was supposed to be impressed—I know because they told me so. They assured me that Chuck's entire case had been very carefully gone over in peer review, but that they couldn't tell me anything that happened because peer review is confidential.

Here is the letter I wrote to Chuck's friend after the first meeting:

> Thank you for pulling together the meeting yesterday. I am determined that change will take place at [the local clinic] so as to prevent others from suffering the tragedy that overtook Chuck and me.
>   My understanding is that two actions were agreed upon:
>
> 1. [The local clinic] will audit the Radiology Department to determine:
>
>   Whether radiologists are truly reading plain films (not just coding them), in accordance with the standards of the American College of Radiology;
>
>   Whether primary physicians and specialists (internists, cardiologists, pulmonologists, family practitioners, pediatricians, etc.) are really looking at all Code 1 films themselves,

2. That within a one-week period, you will e-mail or otherwise let me know of the date of our follow-up meeting as a group, which should be in approximately one month.

We met again in April. At that meeting, the Chief Medical Officer announced that he had developed a plan to figure out once and for all what role the MAFI system was playing. He said that the Code 1 designation was supposed to merely alert referring physicians of a problem needing further workup. He said that the interpretation of the radiologist was wrong: MAFI was *not* designed to allow radiologists to merely screen and code films without reading them—nor to shift the duty of reading them to the nonradiologists.

The CMO said he was very proud of the study he had designed, and of the eminent "outside expert" he had hired to conduct the study. He couldn't describe it in more detail, he said, because it fell under the secret umbrella of peer review. By this time, it was clear to Fred and me that *everything* about Chuck's case fell under that secret umbrella. (Medical peer review is a lot like Las Vegas, in many ways. See the box at the end of this chapter.)

At the next meeting, on May 3, 2004, the study was presented.

The CMO had selected 300 samples of plain chest films which showed a possible malignancy that had never been noted before. From this sample, he had found eighty-two that had been followed by CT scans that confirmed the malignancy. The outside expert he had shown these to had been very impressed that the radiologists had picked up the masses on plain films.

I said that I didn't understand what question this study answered. The problem with Chuck's chest X ray was that it was clearly abnormal but it was *not* followed by a CT scan. What happened, I asked, to the 218 abnormal X rays that were not further investigated? Was Chuck's one of those 218 films?

After a great deal of unhappy discussion, the group finally was able to understand my concerns. I suggested that they substitute an inexpensive study:

1. Pull all the chest X ray reports bearing a Code 1.

2. See if each report included at least one of the following:

   a. An impression of the problem

   b. A differential or specific diagnosis

   c. A suggestion for further studies.

To my gratification, the group agreed to perform this study. But then came time to set the date for the next meeting. It turned out that the only possible date was June 14, 2004.

Chuck had died on June 5, 2003. The statute of limitations for starting a malpractice suit ran out on June 5, 2004. My choices at that moment were:

1. Ignore the legal implications and keep the meeting date for June 14.

2. Obtain an extension of the statute of limitations for another ninety days, running up to September 14.

3. Throw my hands into the air and file a suit immediately.

Nobody at the meeting mentioned the significance of the dates. I was grateful; I knew my options and needed time to think. After twenty-four hours' consideration, it seemed like a slam dunk: file for an extension, keep the date for June 14, and hope for the best.

Unfortunately, I didn't dissect my reasoning; it just seemed like the correct middle road. In fact, however, I was choosing the worst possible route.

I knew I had no intention of suing. My attorney had persuaded me of the folly of doing so. My reason for keeping the threat of suit open was this: I had fallen into the deep black hole of conspiracy theory. Here's what I thought: When Chuck appeared in November 2001 with an obvious terrible cancer *They* went back and saw that *They* had missed it on the previous chest X ray film twenty-two months earlier. *They* were terrified of a malpractice suit. That's why *They* went out of *Their* way to ignore the overwhelming likelihood that this was a treatable malignant thymoma.

It is why *They* seemed to avoid, perversely, looking for a tumor that even a medical student would have suspected.[21] *They* knew that an untreated thymoma would have killed Chuck in three to four months, just as a Cancer of Unknown Primary Site would have done. So *They* decided to let Chuck die with the wrong diagnosis, and nobody would ever know it was wrong.

So, I figured, if there was no threat of a suit, they would have no reason to continue our meetings.

In making this decision, I completely forgot one of Chuck's firmest beliefs: *If you are looking for an explanation of a behavior, and your choice is between conspiracy and incompetence, it is **always** going to be incompetence.*

My bad, as the kids say. Once the Institution was notified that I had filed for an extension, they canceled the June 14 meeting, and no matter what I did I never heard from any of them again.

PEER REVIEW

Another reason why *you* need to monitor your care!

If you sat down and "thought with both hands for a fortnight," you

---

21. Medical students are taught that when a mass appears in the "anterior mediastinum," they should think of four conditions starting with the letter T. This is the kind of memory aid students love. And the first, most common "T" is thymoma. See "Selected Differential Diagnosis of Anterior Mediastinal Masses—the Ts" table within "Photo Quiz: Presistent Cough and Worsening Dyspnea," *American Family Physician*, 71, no. 10 (May 15, 2005).

couldn't come up with a worse concept than peer review as the sole method for preventing and disciplining physician errors in a hospital.

Peer review takes place when a complaint is made about a physician's character, behavior, or actions. The peer review committee then discusses the complaint. In many hospitals, the committee is hand-selected from the more senior physicians, those who feel a sense of "ownership" of the hospital and its workings. The defendant may be an insider with this group, an outsider, or an adversary. This is not supposed to have any effect on the outcome of the Review.

The committee can dismiss the complaint, or it can administer discipline ranging from a friendly rebuke to kicking the physician off the hospital staff, effectively demolishing his or her livelihood and reputation. Most of the criticism of the peer review concept has come from physicians who feel they have been wrongly punished. Many of these cases accuse the committee of using peer review as an instrument to get rid of a competitor, or a whistleblower, or someone they just don't like— perhaps on the grounds of race, religion, ethnicity, or style of dress. Some of these physicians have sued successfully, winning millions of dollars in damages.

Patients who have been injured by the errors of a physician do not have access to the peer review discussions, documents, or findings. Physicians say that if this weren't the case, "peer review would be the inexpensive gathering of evidence for a lawsuit . . . The plaintiffs would just sit back, let the peer reviewers do their thing, then discover what peer review has done and they'd have their case."[22]

The American Medical Association has tried its best to clean up corrupt or sham peer review practices. At the same time, it has thrown itself into preventing states from passing laws that would open the peer review process to others—patients, attorneys, the press.

---

22. James Hilliard, attorney, quoted by Gail Garfinkel Weiss, "Is Peer Review Worth Saving?" *Medical Economics*, February 18, 2005.

No matter how all this sorts out, the underlying problems with peer review will remain:

1. It must be triggered by an error or complaint about something that already has happened.

2. It is adversarial in nature, with a defendant and a jury.

3. There is no mechanism for restitution—no way that an injured patient can receive an apology, explanation, or reimbursement for loss.

4. It adds to the mystique of the "physician brotherhood," in which group loyalty supersedes the interests of the larger society.

SEVENTEEN

Afterthoughts

In the nearly five years since Chuck's diagnosis of malignant thymoma, I have conducted some serious soul-searching, both personally and professionally.

How did we get to this point of medical miracles versus health care chaos?

ENORMOUS CHANGES AT THE LAST MINUTE

Over the last few decades, we've had technological advances coming out our ears. As these new technologies discredit older ones, they require newly trained technicians to make them work, newly educated medical "data" specialists to interpret the diagnostic results, and updated and alert clinical doctors to make the most of those interpretations.

No wonder physicians are swamped: we've got tons more knowledge to assimilate, tons more patients, and tons more paperwork/electronic messaging. Add to this that we are in a technological sticky patch, in which the paper people and the electronic people seem to live on different planets.

MANAGED CARE

For patients, managed care often seems like a dystopian amusement park. It's filled with rides that everybody can take but nobody wants, and rides that everybody wants but nobody can take. There are fine-print regulations and bouncers to enforce them; endless lines of increasingly fed-up patrons, and no actual human being of whom to ask directions

For physicians, managed care is a spider web called a network. My professional duty used to be only to my patient; now it includes a financial duty to my colleagues in my network. I have very little choice of who else or what else (hospital, emergency room) is on my particular network, but clearly we are bonded.

For instance, if I somehow manage to get the network heads to authorize expensive but "uncovered" treatment for a patient, the payment for that treatment comes out of the insurance check that goes to my network. Every physician in the network loses money by it. Even if *I* feel *my* docked check is worth it, my colleague down the road might be put into difficult financial straits.

No wonder the doctor who diagnosed Cancer of Unknown Primary Site did not want to authorize Chuck's out of network care at a cancer center approved by the National Institutes of Health (NIH) Board, the National Cancer Institute (NCI). It is the only not-for-profit organization that investigates and monitors cancer centers for high quality. ("Centers of Excellence" titles are bestowed by insurance plans, for the most part, and standards for excellence vary.)

THE ELEPHANT IN THE ROOM

However, the biggest change is this: Medicine is no longer a profession in which the primary duty of physicians and nurses is to the patient. It is no longer a profession in which it is the duty of physicians to teach those in training.

It's a job.

Physicians and nurses are now the employees of for-profit institutions and/or insurance companies who have to answer to their shareholders. CEOs tend to interpret this responsibility as a duty to make as much money as possible for their shareholders. Their reward comes in the form of salaries and perks.

This short-term profit mentality requires medical and nursing staff to meet a quota of patients seen, X rays read, operations performed. We medical professionals are often penalized, financially and by the withholding of social respect and professional advancement, if our quota isn't met. We are rushed; we must multitask; we become tired and burned out and may fall into short cuts, slipping from the ideal standards of care, despite our best intentions.

Integrity, whether of a person or of an institution, is rarely infinite. It needs bolstering by colleagues and by the way the entire system is conceived and overseen.

A Suggestion

In the Introduction, I bemoaned the absence of the overseer: the person in charge of the big picture. That overseer would check individual documents for internal consistency, related documents for accurate communication, and the whole thing for efficiency and thoroughness.

In the absence of such an omniscient and omnipresent physician overseer, the best person to put in charge of "the big picture" is the patient and his or her loved ones.

Together, they would work as a team, striving for transparency and accountability, resulting in the safety net called physician-patient teamwork.

Transparency

The bulk of this book is about how patients can transform medical reports into documents that they can double-check for omissions, contradictions, and logical lapses. For this task, the more transparent the whole medical process, the better.

Physicians can assist with transparency. Electronic medical records can help, but at this time they have not been perfected. In the meantime, it might help if physicians keep in mind that their reasoning ought to be transparent, even if their words are not. The question to ask oneself, of course, is this: "If I cross out every medical term and substitute the word 'Thing,' will this paragraph still read logically?"

They can also be transparent in identifying themselves and their roles:

- Student doctors and doctors-in-training can introduce themselves as such, wear identifying badges, and sign their dictations with their exact standing: MSC for medical school class, with the year of study; PGR (postgraduate resident) with the year of residency; F/S for Fellow in specialty, with the specialty named.

- Student doctors and doctors-in-training can make clear the name and credentials of their supervising physicians.

Accountability

Physicians should be able to explain and justify their reasoning. Patients can assist this by bringing in the document in question, with their query clearly stated, preferably in writing.

Physicians can help:

- They can make clear in their reports the difference between assumptions and facts.

- They can communicate, and document that communication, with other involved physicians.

- Data doctors can form a habit of including all vital information in each reading, interpretation, and report.

- Doctors who rotate "on call" can ask themselves if the chance assignment of a particular patient forces them to deal with a diagnosis out of their realm of comfort. If so, they should arrange to transfer care to a different physician.

- Doctors can treat "diagnoses of exclusion" and "non-diagnoses"[23] as challenges for further consideration, rather than as conclusions.

- Supervising physicians can truly critique student documents, marking corrections in ink, and remember that their signature counts as a validation of whatever they sign.

MORAL OF THE STORY

I know how well this can work.

Pediatricians have always occupied a special role in medicine. We are always communicating with the loving adults who care for our young patients. For that reason, we are trained, both by senior doctors and by the parents of our patients, to be as clear, transparent, and accountable as possible. Many of the non-medically trained adults we talk with are highly sophisticated. They already review their children's medical reports, and are not at all shy about asking us questions and calling us to account. They go online to check on us, and to talk with each other and us.

Also, pediatricians tend to communicate very freely with each other— at least in my own thirty-year experience. And we tend not to use medicalese a whole lot; we get out of the habit by talking with six-year-olds. We call a red throat a red throat, not an erythematous pharynx, euphonious as it may be.

So I know this can work. I hope we can make it do so for all of us.

---

23. A non-diagnosis is one that consists merely of symptoms, signs, or study reports. Examples: "chronic headache," "limp," "enlarged heart," or "anemia." There is no cause identified.

PART FOUR

Workbook

INTRODUCTION:

Who Needs This Work?

You don't need to delve thoroughly into a chart if you have no reason to worry. If that's your situation, I suggest you merely form the habit of obtaining your medical documents as they accrue in the future, checking them quickly for red flags and filing them away.

The crucial reason to investigate your chart boils down to one thing only: You feel the need to be the person in charge and in control, and you are aware that nobody else has really taken that on.

In my view, here are pressing reasons to perform a true excavation and analysis of your chart:

- You have a "diagnosis of exclusion" or other uncertain diagnosis, and are not sure exactly what other possible diagnoses are being considered, why they are being considered, and how they are being excluded.

- You are at risk for a malignancy or other condition, and receive routine examinations and studies designed to screen for it.

- You have been given a clean bill of health but continue to have ongoing or increasing symptoms.

- You have been diagnosed with a serious condition that is rare.

- You have been diagnosed with a condition not usually found in someone of your age, or gender, or race, or history of exposure

- You have looked up your diagnosis (say, on www.wrongdiagnosis. com) and the description of that diagnosis does not fit your symptoms.

- Your faith in those directing your medical care has been shaken for any reason whatsoever.

- You have an insurance problem.

Of course, you are perfectly free to tackle your chart for no reason in particular. It doesn't mean you are masochistic or weird; you may just want to get better acquainted with what your physician thinks about you. You might well run into pleasant surprises:

"This delightful gentleman appearing much younger than his stated age"

"This bright and sunny six-year-old girl"

"This highly intelligent and articulate mother of five"

At any rate, the following workbook is designed to help you organize your approach, whatever your reason. It follows the same strategy I used with Chuck's records, as described in Part I, The Dicey Diagnosis.

EIGHTEEN

The Case of Lily the Cheerleader

This is a true story of a girl I'll call Lily, a story in which everything went right, but which was threatened with many possible glitches—small, common problems that could have endangered the life of my teenage patient. If that *had* happened, the danger could have been spotted and circumvented by Lily's mother.

It is the Friday afternoon before I leave on vacation, and I'm behind schedule. So it's after four o'clock when I head toward the fifteen-year-old girl in exam room 12.

Fortunately, I've known Lily since her birth, and I know she and her mother will forgive my tardiness. Before I go into the room, I check my tablet-sized WiFi computer. Here is my medical assistant's recap of Lily's chief complaint: "Tired and cough; had to miss cheerleading practice." Knowing Lily, I suspect that the only reason she agreed to a doctor's visit was the missed cheer practice.

"Cheer," she tells me now, as she does at each visit, "is my *life!*"

"And she refuses to wear a hat," her mother chimes in, at which Lily rolls her eyes. "No wonder she's coughing. I want her to get an X ray!"

I doubt that's necessary. Lily probably has "cheerleader's cough," a slight irritation from high-pitched screaming. I myself have heard Lily lead cheers.

I start to examine Lily in my usual sequence: ears, nose, throat, chest (the sounds of a little pneumonia, or irritation called pneumonitis, on the right side, nothing to get excited about), heart, lymph nodes. Uh oh. My hands freeze in place. Lily has a firm unmovable lump the size of a grape peeking over her collarbone. A lymph node. It is called a "sentinel node" because it isn't a normal part of the healthy body. Often it is the first sign of news, usually bad news. *Teenager, fatigue, supraclavicular lymph node, abnormal lung exam: the classic presentation of Hodgkin's lymphoma.*

I tell myself not to jump to conclusions. Radiology is about to close, but I persuade them to stay open another half hour for Lily's chest X ray.

The report is on the following page.

Read it as you did the reports in the chapters about Chuck: Simply cross out the words that are unfamiliar and substitute the word "thing" or "thingy." Then concentrate on the ones that you understand. The familiar words tell you the story clearly: Lily has a *mass* in her chest. We all know that's not good. She needs to get a CT of the chest and also a consultation with a specialist. It sounds as if her illness is likely to be serious.

I send Lily to the emergency room at the pediatric hospital.[24] The emergency room doctor admits her to the hospital where indeed she is soon diagnosed with Hodgkin's lymphoma, a cancer of the lymph system. It is the earliest stage, Stage 1, the best possible news in this situation. The cancer is limited to her chest, and her chance of a true cure is high: 75 to 95 percent.

A scary diagnosis indeed, but a diagnostic process that went without a glitch. Glitches would have meant delays, and might have meant a more advanced cancer and a much darker prognosis for Lily.

---

24. I cannot admit her directly because of the shortage of hospital beds and nurses. Every admission must be okayed by the emergency room staff.

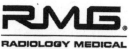

RADIOLOGY MEDICAL GROUP, INC.

ENCINITAS IMAGING CENTER
477 N. EL CAMINO REAL, SUITE A102
ENCINITAS, CA 92024
PHONE: (619) 849-XRAY (849-9729)

PATIENT NAME   ACCOUNT NO MEDICAL RECORD NUMBER

AT THE REQUEST OF DATE OF BIRTH AGE/SEX DATE OF SERVICE
LAURA NATHANSON M.D. 17/M
  EL CAMINO REAL
SUITE B-105
ENCINITAS, CA 92024

CENTRALIZED NUMBERS
PHN: (619) 849-XRAY (849-9729)
FAX: (619) 849-4RMG (849-4764)

DIAGNOSTIC RADIOLOGY
OFFICES

FIRST & LAUREL
IMAGING CENTER
2466 First Avenue
San Diego, CA 92101-1492
FAX (619) 696-7859

SCRIPPS MERCY HEALTHCARE
Department of Radiology
4077 Fifth Avenue
San Diego, CA 92103-2180
FAX: (619) 543-1076

MERCY MAGNETIC
IMAGING CENTER
4077 Fifth Avenue
San Diego, CA 92103-2180
FAX: (619) 543-1076

ENCINITAS
IMAGING CENTER
477 N. El Camino Real,
Suite A102
Encinitas, CA 92024-1329
FAX: (760) 632-5369

ADMINISTRATIVE OFFICE
3366 Fifth Avenue
P. O. Box 34307
San Diego, CA 92163-4307
FAX: (619) 294-8399

Check out our website
radiologybyrmg.com

PROCEDURE: TWO-VIEW CHEST

COMPARISON: None.

FINDINGS: There is a 5.0 x 8.0 cm right paratracheal well-circumscribed mass, apparently located in the right anterior mediastinum. It is confluent with the right superior hilum.

In addition, increased interstitial markings are seen extending from the right hilum in to the right lower lobe, suggesting an interstitial pneumonitis.

The left lung is clear. No left hilar adenopathy.

CONCLUSION:

1. **Right paratracheal mass with right lower lobe pneumonitis.**
2. **Thymic mass could also explain the right paratracheal findings.**

RECOMMENDATIONS:

Pulmonary consultation and chest CT.

Thank you for referring this patient,

clf
Dictated: 1/18/00; Typed: 1/19/00

"WHAT IF" SCENARIO: GLITCHES IN DIAGNOSIS

Suppose:

- I don't mention the possible scary diagnosis in the office. I don't want to terrify Lily and her mom, I am not positive of the diagnosis, and I am all too aware of the resentment some patients feel on the announcement of bad news—a sort of "blame the messenger" phenomenon. I will let the hospital specialists present the problem; they are used to doing so, and will have answers about treatment. Besides, I am due to leave for Baja at 5 A.M.

- The radiologist who reads the chest X ray dictates an incomplete report that omits the "Conclusion" and the "Recommendations." (It's Friday night, after 5 P.M., and he's got theater tickets.)

- The emergency room computer isn't set up to receive electronic transmissions of X ray pictures, or images, from outside X ray departments. It can only receive the typewritten reports of the radiologist. Thus, once Lily is in the hospital, there's no way for her doctors to examine the chest X ray itself; only the truncated report.

- The very young ER doctor reads the incomplete chest X ray report. What is she to make of it? The term "well-circumscribed" seems to be reassuring, even though a mass is mentioned. Certainly, if there were a tumor, wouldn't the radiologist have said so? It's probably a classic description of something innocent (maybe a perfectly normal thymus gland) that the brand-new doctor ought to know, but doesn't—and she doesn't want to ask. To be safe, she decides to admit Lily and let the staff on the ward figure out the chest X ray business.

- On the infectious disease ward, Lily is assigned to a medical student, as is customary at this teaching hospital. He thinks that the offhandedness of the X ray report plus the fact that the emergency room doctor didn't mention the mass means that it is unimportant.

- He writes a report designed to impress his supervising doctor, with a complete discussion of pneumonitis, its common and rare causes. As a finishing touch, he includes footnoted references to the literature, gleaned by Googling.

- The senior doctor overseeing the medical student skims the student's report and is extremely impressed by the footnotes. She doesn't pause to read the X ray interpretation. Why bother? This is clearly an *overly* conscientious third-year who jumps all over the slightest abnormality—even a little pneumonitis! Unworried, and overwhelmed by a dozen other "really sick" patients, the senior doctor endorses the student's conclusion of a minor infectious disease.

- On antibiotics, Lily seems somewhat better by the next morning and is discharged: The hospital "needs her bed."

- Hours before her discharge, I have left for my vacation surfing in Baja, and am completely out of reach for two weeks. When I return, there are so many reports to review that I don't get to Lily's, which alas has become lost at the bottom of my priority list. After all, I think, she's in the hands of specialists by now.

- Lily, determined to return to cheer practice, hides her symptoms of fatigue, night sweats, and chest pain from her parents.

- When Lily shows up back in the emergency room five weeks later with widespread Hodgkin's and a poor prognosis, everyone is shocked and appalled.

Lily's Mother Intervenes

This nightmare version of Lily's diagnosis didn't happen. But it could have, all too easily.

Let us suppose that the nightmare scenario does occur. Lily is admitted to the hospital, treated overnight for a lung infection, and discharged on Saturday morning.

But Lily's mother is not happy. Lily isn't acting right. She looks pale. Her sheets are soaked with sweat in the morning. Her usually animated cell-phone conversations consist of inarticulate noises. She needs a nap Saturday and Sunday.

Now, Lily's mother, as Lily frequently and offensively observes, is *"not a doctor and has had no medical training whatsoever!"* But she knows her daughter, and she trusts her own much-tried instincts.

The first thing her mother thinks of is pregnancy, and then drugs. On Monday, she calls the pediatric office and is told that I have run away to Baja for two weeks. She doesn't know my partners very well, and decides to hold off calling again until I return. *But she doesn't stop there! Something, she is sure, isn't right.*

Lily's mother:

1. Obtains a copy of the medical records of Lily's brief hospital stay.

2. Reads the admitting note by the medical student and notices that there is no mention of pregnancy or drugs. ("What is the matter with these people?" she thinks. "Don't they read the newspapers?")

3. Finds the (incomplete) chest X ray report and sees the word "MASS." Her eyebrows go up. Nobody told her anything about a mass in Lily's chest! What what what what what is going on here!

She calls my pediatric office and in outrage demands to speak to my partner. My partner looks at the chest X ray image and report on his computer and is horrified. He breaks the news that Lily needs an immediate CT of the chest and readmission to the hospital. Within forty-eight hours, Lily is diagnosed with stage 1 Hodgkin's disease, and starts treatment.

When I return from Baja, I find that Lily is no longer my patient; she has transferred to my partner. I hear the story and feel as awful as you can imagine, send an abject note of apology to Lily's mother and flowers to Lily.

As happy an ending as possible. Lily gets quickly and accurately diagnosed and treated. I get to apologize sincerely and send up prayers of gratitude. The radiologist, emergency room doctor, medical student, and supervising physician all are galvanized to repent and reform. Nobody gets sued. Lily's cheer squad comes and entertains the entire oncology ward.

Lily's mother (once Lily's excellent prognosis is determined) gets to savor her own successful intervention, Lily's admiration and gratitude, and my humble atonement. She is indeed the hero of her daughter's life.

NINETEEN

First, Get Your Chart

STRATEGY SUMMARY

I. Physician Narratives

Create a stack → Sort each stack → Pull most recent or →
of Physician chronologically, important Physician
Narratives and most recent on top. Narrative. Locate
a stack of Data Make sure they are section dealing with
Reports all yours! "Assessment,"
"Diagnosis," etc.

Replace each → Delete sentences → Circle all →
medical term now rendered Scary/Uncertain
with word "Thing." meaningless. words or terms.

Is there a Scary → Look for Fuzzy → See if a Study could
possibility that Logic—a "thought" clarify the true mean-
has not been with two or more ing. If so, find its Data
excluded? Write possible and opposite Report.
it in Workbook. meanings. Write all
versions in Workbook.

→ Finally: Enter in the Workbook all possible diagnoses given by any physician.

II. Data Reports

A. Imaging studies: X ray, ultrasound, CT, MRI, Barium swallow or enema: anything performed/read by Radiologist.

- Check "Conclusion" section as above for Scary, Uncertain, and Fuzzy Logic

- Check entire document for completeness

- Enter in the Workbook all suggested diagnoses.

B. Pathology Reports

- Is the tissue biopsied the correct tissue?

- Is the sample stated to be adequate?

- Circle all medical entities tested for.

- Write circled terms in Workbook.

- Match the "Possible Diagnoses" list against the "Tested For" list. Were all diagnoses considered?

FIRST, GET YOUR CHART

When Lily's mother couldn't reach me, she went and got Lily's chart. Yep, just like that.

You are entitled, even urged, to obtain your own medical records, or those of a dependent family member or friend. This entitlement and encouragement comes to you direct from Washington D.C.

In April 2003, a federal act came into effect called HIPAA: the Health Information Portability and Accountability Act. This act decrees that your access to your own chart is a personal right of every American. This federal law overrides state laws that forbid such access, as well as any dissenting personal opinions of doctors and their staffs.

FIND YOUR RECORDS

Your entire chart may be filed in one location, such as your primary care doctor's office or the medical records department at one of the many full-service clinics, such as Kaiser Permanente.

However, sometimes the records are scattered. If you have had care for any significant problem at a different office, clinic, or have been admitted to the hospital, that part of your records may still be at that location, and may not be included in your most recent chart at your primary care doctor's office. If that is the case, you will need to apply for your old records to each office or hospital at which they were generated.

There is no state, medical board, or federal clearinghouse that contains all medical records, or all immunizations, or all of anything, as far as I can see.

JUST ASK FOR THE CHART

Start with the patient's own physician's office. Even if the patient's care has been dispersed, there is a pretty good chance his or her own doctor has been sent the out-of-office records.

Ask the person at the front desk (the receptionist) how to obtain a Medical Records Release form. Someone in the office is in charge of such forms.

Make out the form to have the records released to you. If the records you are requesting are yours, you only need to sign the form and show photo ID. Most of the time, this is also all you need when you ask for the records of your children under the age of eighteen. If you are asking for someone else's records (a spouse, adult friend, or family member, for instance) you will be asked for that person's written, documented consent. Some offices may ask that the consent be witnessed or even notarized.

The form asks you if you want the complete records or only part of them—hospital reports, say, or surgical procedures. Even though it increases your copying costs, it is safest to ask for the entire record. Some of the most important materials (hospital discharges or specialists' reports) may have been misfiled under sections such as "insurance documents" or "informed consent copies." If so, they may not be identified and will be missing from your copy.

Moreover, having the entire chart in your possession is a protection in the event that legal steps are taken. It means that you can document whether a correction to a report was made before or after the date you came into possession of the chart. It is a felony to falsify information in a medical chart.

The staff person checks your ID, takes the filled-out form, and tells you when the copy of the records will ready for you to pick up. The copying fee varies from place to place, and is determined by the number of pages to copy.

Only rare, special circumstances should prevent you from obtaining a copy of your patient's entire chart.

PICKING THEM UP

The copied medical records may come to you in any of several kinds of bundles, depending on the size of the record, the secretarial skills of the office, and its technical sophistication—paper chart versus electronic medical record (EMR) versus paper-EMR hybrid.

Your paper chart may consist of a pile of papers spilling out of their encircling rubber bands with no dividers to separate the different categories. More happily, you might get a neatly stacked pile of papers with some kind of divider—a piece of cardboard, with or without an

PICKING UP THE MEDICAL RECORD

- Bring along a sturdy box that holds $8^1/_2 \times 11$ papers, with at least a two-inch depth. If you anticipate a very lengthy record, bring more boxes.

- Keep the pages in order! Even if they seem to be all tumbled together, chances are good that many are where they're supposed to be.

- Keep the receipt for the medical records. If any legal proceedings ensue, you'll want to have a record of the date you received them. This will help to make sure that nobody can make changes to the record with falsified dates.

identifier—separating categories (in theory, anyway). Best scenario: A stack of papers in a binder, complete with dividers.

Unless the patient is a young baby whose medical life is recorded entirely electronically, you may find yourself with a combined paper-EMR chart. The EMR part of the chart may be printouts, a CD of the EMR, or an e-mail transmission directly to you. I strongly advise you to obtain a complete copy of that paper chart as well as the print-out or electronic transmission of the entire EMR. Do this even if you are told that the paper chart is "in storage." Ask for it to be retrieved.

Now that you have your chart in hand, it is time to put it in order.

TWENTY

Four Crucial Stacks

A Mindless Task

A medical record is a lot like a meatloaf. It can omit what you might think would be crucial ingredients (such as meat) and include others (such as tofu) that seem incongruous, and still be called a medical record (meatloaf). Sometimes everything is jumbled together; sometimes it is carefully layered, or rolled up like a jelly roll.

Lily's mother was lucky. The chart for Lily's overnight admission was only seven pages long: the one-page chest X ray report, a one-page emergency room note, a two-page admitting note signed by the medical student and supervising doctor, a discharge note, one page of medication and lab orders, and one page of nurses' notes.

However, some charts are really big and/or messy.

Even if it is tidy, organized, and has everything in labeled sections, you will have to tame the record for your present purposes, because about 90 percent of it is irrelevant to your interests. You need to discard all that irrelevant material. **What you want to have left is the meat in the meatloaf: the indelible brainprint of how somebody is thinking.**

Every document you save will reveal:

- The thinker's interpretation (or Conclusion, Assessment, Discussion, Comments)

- The thinker's recommendation (or Suggestions, Plan, Other Studies)

- The identity, credentials, and rank of the person doing the thinking

There are four categories of documents bearing this information. The first three categories are narratives generated by clinical care doctors. The last category consists of reports on studies, made by data-providing doctors.

1. Primary care doctor's dictated reports on office visits

2. Hospital admissions (history and physical)

3. Consultations from specialists

4. Typed reports from the data-providing doctors

Let us hope that all of these categories are correctly filed, in correctly labeled sections of the chart, but don't count on it. In order to focus all our attention on this important material, you have to have it in good order. This means you can't just pull out each set of documents from its labeled section and assume that you're done. You need to go through each of the sections, removing duplicates, correcting the misfiled, lining up two-or-more-paged documents in the correct reading order, and checking for missing pages.

That's not all. Then you need to go through the rest of the chart, looking for documents that have straggled away from their home section. An important hospital admission might be stuffed into the section labeled "correspondence" or "labs" or "insurance."

Fortunately, you don't have to puzzle over every single page. Look for papers that:

- are typed, not handwritten[25]

- contain at the end of the report a section marked "Discussion" or a synonym, such as "Impression," "Assessment," "Problems"

- bear a signature line or lines, usually at the bottom of the last page of the document

With the four categories extracted, and the stragglers rescued, everything else can be placed (unsorted and unread) into a box. It is unlikely but possible that one or more of these discards may turn out to be important, so don't throw away the box.

Creating the four crucial stacks with some care now will make your task of reading and analysis much more focused. So bear with me for a bit more dusty, paper cut–laden scut work.

Line the stacked documents of each category in chronological order, with the oldest on the bottom and the latest on top. When you encounter a multipage document, staple the pages together in order as if you were reading it as a letter.

As you go along, check to make sure that the papers are all really yours, and not somebody else's. Check the name, date of birth, and gender on each page of each report. You may find that your chart contains portions of somebody else's chart, often for no apparent reason. I have known people to become strangely attached to this phantom chartmate. Try to resist.[26]

Then start numbering the individual pages from the oldest to the

---

25. Some psychiatrists and psychologists prefer to handwrite reports. I do not deal with mental illness in this book, however.

26. Sometimes there's a clear reason for such chart invasion. My patient Spencer Taylor is a boy, and my patient Spenser Taylor is a girl. They've never met, but their misfiled reports have merged their charts into a hermaphrodite. How many practices have both a Matthew Owen and an Owen Matthew? Or an Emily Wilkins age two and an Emily Wilkins age fourteen? Or three Lesley Hamptons, all born in the same month and year?

newest, so that new records will have the highest numbers; that way, you can continue to add documents as they are generated.

Finally, remove from the bottom of the stacks any documents more than two years old. They are unlikely to be relevant now, but don't throw them into the discard box; label and keep them in a more dignified storage arrangement.

You now have reduced the chart to manageability and relevance. Once we stop sneezing and our fingertips stop bleeding, we can move on to the next chapter, in which we will have to turn on our brains.

===

TWENTY-ONE

Clinical Physician Narratives

The first order of business is to examine the physician narratives. There are four sets of worksheets in this chapter. Fill them out for every physician narrative you examine.

1. Anxious alliance of scary and uncertain

2. Fuzzy logic

3. Non-diagnosis

4. Summary of clarifying studies

Worksheet 1: The Anxious Alliance (Scary + Uncertain)

Document Date: Title: Dictated by: Supervising Physician & Title:		
Page #	Scary Word or Diagnosis	Uncertainty Term or Diagnosis

Worksheet 1: The Anxious Alliance *(continued)*

Was diagnosis both scary and uncertain?	Is there a study that could provide certainty? What is it?	Is there a plan for obtaining that study?

Worksheet 2: Fuzzy Logic

Document Date: Title: Dictated by: Supervising Physician:		
Page #	Fuzzy Logic Sentence	List of Possible Versions of Fuzzy Logic Sentence
Scary versions of sentence	What are scary possibilities of rewritten sentence?	Is there a study that could clarify the illogic?

Worksheet 2: Fuzzy Logic *(continued)*

Study That Could Clarify	Performed: Result	Plan for Study

There are several kinds of non-diagnoses:

- Differential diagnosis: A list of possibilities, often in no particular order.

- Idiopathic: Cause not identified and not expected to be identified

- Unknown etiology: Cause not identified, but still might be identified

- Non-Diagnosis:

  - Symptom instead of cause: "arthritis"; "chronic abdominal pain"; "recurrent headaches"; "failure to thrive"

  - Physical finding instead of cause: "jaundice"; "enlarged spleen;" "dehydration"

  - Lab or imaging finding instead of a cause: "anemia"; "mass"; "enlarged heart."

Worksheet 3: Non-Diagnosis

Document Date: Title: Dictated by: Supervising Physician:			
Differential Diagnosis	List of Entities Considered	Scary Possibility?	Study to Clarify
Idiopathic Diagnosis or Unknown Etiology	List of Excluded Causes		Study Performed to Clarify
Non-Diagnosis	Differential Diagnosis Suggested?		If so, study performed to clarify?

Worksheet 4: Summary of All Clarifying Studies Listed

Study	Performed on This Date	Scheduled to Be Performed	Not Done or Planned

Worksheet 1: Pulling Relevant Data

Return to your Summary at the end of Workbook 1. Consult your fourth critical stack to see whether you have a clarifying data report.

Scary/Uncertain Possibility:	Data Report That Could Clarify	Do you have that report in your stack?
Fuzzy Logic Rewritten Sentences That Are Scary:	Data Report that Could Clarify	Do you have that report in your stack?
Differential Diagnosis Lists	Data Report That Could Clarify	Do you have that report in your stack?
"Non-Diagnosis" Entities	Study That Could Clarify	Do you have that report in your stack?

TWENTY-TWO

Data Reports

You now have an idea whether studies have been done, or are still needed to disprove (or confirm) a scary possible diagnosis. Your next task is to see whether you have a copy of the study interpretation. The task of judging the quality of the interpretations comes later.

All your study reports should be in the hitherto untouched fourth stack. Pull out all the study reports you have flagged in the last chapter on clinical physician narratives. Start by pulling out the imaging studies and sorting them by type: plain X ray, CT, MRI, ultrasound, and so on.

Then pull out the pathology (cytopathology) reports (consultations).

The pile you have left will contain "Procedure" reports—studies of body processes while they are going on. These include EEGs (brain-waves), EKGs (heart electricity), and anything else that isn't included in imaging studies and pathology.

There are two kinds of data reports I have *not* included in this workbook, nor indeed in the work as a whole. They're another whole book's worth.

1. Laboratory values: Laboratory test results on blood, urine, etc. are generated by technology and transmitted by computer printout.

2. Investigative Procedures performed on one's living, breathing self to determine how various organs are functioning. These include EKG, EEG, and "endoscopies."

Missing Data Reports

Go over the tables you have just completed and flag the documents missing from your data stack.

Type of Study	Could Clarify This Question	Any possibility study was performed but report is missing?

If you are almost certain the study was indeed performed, and you believe that the clarification is important, you have two options. One is to go through all the discarded papers of the chart, looking for it. The other is to make a separate, specific request for a copy of the report. To do this, you would need to know where the study was performed, and ideally the name of the ordering physician.

TWENTY-THREE

Imaging Study Reports

Separate out the imaging study reports—anything performed in the radiology department. List them all in the table below:

Type of Imaging Study	Date of Study	Radiologist	Ordering Clinical Physician

You have three important questions to answer about each report:

1. Does the radiologist understand the big issue(s) and address them?

2. Is the interpretation complete?

3. Is it unambiguous?

It is, I believe, easiest to start with Question 2, because all it requires is a checklist. So I suggest you start here:

QUESTION 2: HOW COMPLETE IS THIS STUDY REPORT?

Study: Date Performed: Date Dictated:		
Radiologist:		
Ordering Clinical Physician:		
Is the following guideline addressed in this report?	Yes, No, or Implied	If implied, what is implication?
Reason for study		
Factors limiting accuracy		
Previous study for comparison		
Relevant clinical issues		
Detailed assessment of findings, with measurements, locations, shape		
Incidental/unrelated findings		
Interpretation, not just repetition of findings		
Definite diagnosis		
Differential list of possible diagnoses		
Suggestions for further studies or actions		

QUESTION 1: QUALITY OF REPORT

Does the radiologist address the big issue(s)?

There are two ways the radiologist could do this. He could state the big issue under "Reason for Study" or similar heading. Or he could assume that the big issue is obvious and understood, and answer it in the Interpretation /Diagnosis/ Suggestions for further studies.

If neither of these is evident, the answer to this question is No.

Is the report complete? If it is not, is this an understandable omission of something unnecessary, or a lapse that could cause problems?

Very likely to cause problems:

- Omission of a definitive or differential diagnosis

- The "Interpretation" merely repeats the "Findings" or is absent entirely

- A differential diagnosis without suggested further studies

Unlikely to be a serious problem:

- If "Previous Study for Comparison" is blank, assume that no study was available. In that case, however, bear in mind that therefore the radiologist should make no assumptions of what is a new finding or what was preexisting. If such an assumption is made, this is a possibly dangerous omission.

- If "Relevant Clinical Issues" is omitted, but the other sections in Question 1 are answered, this is likely to be because the radiologist assumed that the relevant clinical issues were obvious. Not likely to be serious.

QUESTION 3: IS THE INTERPRETATION AMBIGUOUS?

An ambiguous interpretation is one that doesn't explain the findings. There are two possible reasons for ambiguity: The first one is that the situation itself is ambiguous; there is more than one possible diagnosis.

If this is the case, there should be a "differential diagnosis" and, often, suggestions for further studies.

The second one is that a flaw in the interpretation or logic produces ambiguity. Read the interpretation carefully, looking for fuzzy logic.

Study: Date: Radiologist: Institution			
Big Issue	Definitive Diagnosis	Differential Diagnosis	Not Addressed

Is the Interpretation Complete?

Report	Dangerous Omissions

Is the Diagnosis Ambiguous Due to Fuzzy Logic?

Report	Diagnosis	Fuzzy Logic

ACTION

If any of your answers to questions 1, 2, or 3 are worrisome, take the report plus your worksheets to your primary care physician or to the specialist who ordered the study. Ask for clarification and write it down in the following chart:

Report	Worrisome Entry	Clarification	Consultant Clarifying

TWENTY-FOUR

Pathology Study Reports

Before you take this on, I suggest you review Chapter 7, Red Flags: Pathology Reports.

Tissue	Pathologist	Date	Ordered by	
First Opinion or Consultation	If consultation, who was first pathologist?		What were findings of first pathologist?	
Method of Obtaining	Fine Needle or Swab	Open (surgery)	Other	Not Stated
Sample Size				
Condition of Sample				

Differential Diagnosis Mentioned Anywhere in Your Records	Suggested by (Primary Doctor, Specialist, Radiologist, Pathologist)	Tested for in Biopsy	Not in List of Tests

Definite Diagnosis or "Most Likely Possibility"	No Fuzzy Logic	Fuzzy Logic

Summarize Your Findings of Any Worrisome Features

Report	Method	Missing Diagnosis	Fuzzy Logic

TWENTY-FIVE

Pulling It All Together

In this chapter, you will figure out where any danger points may be and what your options are for dealing with them. The final worksheet will help you to clarify the data you have collected in the previous chapters. When you complete it, you should have an idea of whether your chart has revealed something significant that needs fixing, what it would take to fix it, and the best person to do the fixing.

Summary of Your Physician Narrative Worksheets

Study or Data Report That Could Clarify Fuzzy Logic	Performed and Clarified	Performed But Not Clarified	Not Performed

Summary of Your Physician Narrative Worksheets
(continued)

Study or Data Report That Could Clarify Non-Diagnosis	Performed and Clarified	Performed But Not Clarified	Not Performed

Summary of Your Imaging Studies Worksheets

As described in Chapter 23, it's best to try to get clarification on these data reports before summarizing your entire chart.

Report	Worrisome Entry	Clarification	Consultant Clarifying

Pathology Reports Worksheet

Report	Missing Sample Description as Adequate	Missing Investigation of Suggested Diagnosis	Fuzzy Logic

"Who's in Charge Here?" Worksheet

Diagnosis Being Treated	ABMS Certified in Appropriate Specialty	Daily Function as Stated on Business Card or on Hospital or Individual Web Site	Appropriate Experience for Particular Condition: Yes/No/Unknown

Your Game Plan

Problem	What It Would Take to Fix It	Best Medical Source for Help

OPTIONS

If you find an active problem, keep in mind that your goal is to get the problem fixed as quickly as possible. It is not to place blame or be confrontational.

I strongly suggest that you bring your work sheets and the relevant documents of the medical record along to any encounter. It is most helpful to write down in full sentences your understanding of the nature of the problem. In doing so, do not pin blame; merely describe what the evidence shows. Take the letter with you, and if the encounter becomes emotional, stop conversing and instead read out loud.

You have six avenues for getting the problem fixed:

1. Address the physicians directly responsible for your concerns.

2. Seek help from the hospital (or other institution):

   a. The chief of the department

   b. The head of the peer review committee or the quality control committee

   c. The hospital ombudsman

3. Get a second opinion, ideally at a different institution. (See the appendix on managed care.)

4. Call your insurance company. Most of the large ones have a public relations staff trained to deal with complaints. Make sure that you have a clear, relatively brief statement to make, and that you do not blame the insurance company for any errors you perceive. If you can get one of the staff on your side, you may luck into rapid resolution of your problem.

5. If the problem is related to cancer diagnosis and treatment, you can try calling one of the NCI designated[27] cancer centers, and asking for advice. This is one way for you to address your own physician about the issue: once you have spoken with a cutting-edge expert on a particular kind of cancer, you can ask your own physician to discuss your case with that expert.

6. If you have tried to take action and have met with resistance, or if you have had assistance but you are still given a diagnosis of

---

27. See p. 116.

exclusion or other "dicey diagnosis," you have the following actions to choose from:

a. Call your insurance company and press for a second opinion.

b. If you are on an HMO, try to change your primary care provider. This usually can be done at the first of each month. Change to a PCP who is in an IPA that covers hospitals or specialists with better ratings for treating your particular problem. See the appendix about health care plans.

c. If you are on a PPO, find the most expert physician in the field of your illness, regardless of whether he or she is in your network. If necessary, be prepared to travel and to pay a big co-pay to find that expert.

d. Go online to: www.wrongdiagnosis.com and read everything relevant to your problem.

TOO LATE TO FIX

If the problem has already brought consequences that cannot be reversed, but you want to make sure that it is addressed and prevented from happening again, your best choice is likely to be contacting the Joint Commission on Accreditation of Health Care Organizations (JCAHO). Make sure you have all the specific information with names, addresses, and dates. Remember that you must report within a year of the incident.

Phone: 800-994-6610 weekdays, 8:30 A.M. to 5:00 P.M. central time

E-mail: no more than two pages sent to **complaint@jcaho.org**

Download a complaint form at **www.jcaho.org,** click on "General Public" and then on "Go to Report a Complaint."

You could also file a complaint with the state licensing board in your state—medicine or osteopathic. Ask your search engine, or call information.

As for litigation, publicity, or "going to the top" to complain, you already know my experience with that. But every case is different.

I suggest you do not bother with state "medical societies," as these are simply lobbying groups for physicians.

Managed Care

PART 1: CAN YOU ESCAPE IT ALTOGETHER?

Managed care is so filled with red tape and traps that I suggest you start by deciding whether you might be able to bypass the whole scene.

You Can Bypass Managed Care If

- You are rich. You can either pay cash for everything or choose an "indemnity plan." These plans have a high deductible before they kick in. As for co-payments, they pay 80 percent of what they deem to be a "reasonable" fee for each service. You pay 20 percent plus anything that goes over the "reasonable" fee.

- You have another form of payment: military, Medicare, Medicaid. In this case, your care is paid for under federal law, and you can either choose everything you want, or the choices are already made for you.

- You are at very low risk for requiring medical care over the next year and can choose either the cheapest HMO offered, or a Health Savings Account (HSA). HSAs are new and evolving, and I have decided not to discuss them here.

Very Low Risk

If all of the following apply, and will continue to apply over the following year, both to you *and to your dependents*, you may consider yourself very low risk.

- Age 35 or younger

- Not pregnant, no possibility of becoming pregnant

- No dependents who are over the age of 18, and there is no possibility of acquiring such dependents by birth, marriage, adoption, or other means

- Nobody with a condition requiring specialist care within the last five years

- Nobody with a condition that has required hospitalization in the last five years

- Nobody with a condition known to have remissions and exacerbations (eating disorders, multiple sclerosis, etc.)

- Nobody with a condition requiring prescription medication (including birth control pills)

- No family history of sudden unexpected death or of any serious disease before age 50

- No known risk for a serious genetic disease

- Nobody with lifestyle risks: seriously overweight; habit or addiction (tobacco, alcohol, drugs); risky pastimes: contact sports, accident-prone activities, sexual adventuring, road rage, etc. If you think something is a risk, I'm sure it is; and I cannot name them all.

- No sneaking suspicion that you've all been much too lucky, medically speaking

If you really are in a very low risk category, congratulations. Just remember this: things can change. Tomorrow you may fall madly in love with someone who has five children, takes three expensive daily medications, and just loves snowboarding—and who needs to be put on your insurance plan.

My only additional, nonmedical advice to you risk-free, carefree young things: make sure you have disability insurance, especially if you are the primary breadwinner, or if you have had expensive education and training for a high-paying profession, or still have student loans pending.

PART 2: PPOs, HMOs, AND POSs

Before you sort through the HMOs, PPOs, and POSs available to you, keep in mind the important differences among these three kinds of managed care.

A Short Review of Managed Care

Back before there were "networks" and "medical groups" and "IPAs," insurance companies ran the whole show. They were gigantic and their power was undisputed, sort of like dinosaurs. They were able to kick doctors and hospitals off their provider lists at will, and recontract their services for less money.

In an attempt to have some power, physicians formed groups, which could bargain with the insurance firms. They negotiate a contract that says, "We'll take money from you (a certain amount for each of your insurees who enrolls with us) and use it to pay for medical care for our patients. In return, we will 'assume risk'—that is, take over the decisions about care for these patients."

And that, my dears, was the birth of managed care.

Like the insurance firms, these groups are interested in controlling medical costs. They can't increase their income; the insurance plans are too powerful for them to negotiate a larger sum of money. So they keep costs down by imposing restrictions: which doctors a patient can see; what hospital they can go to; what specialists to be referred to; what "durable equipment" (such as wheelchairs) will be paid for, and under what conditions.

The less a plan costs (in monthly premiums and copayments), the fewer choices it gives you in doctors, emergency rooms, hospitals, lab tests, imaging studies, and prescription medications. Conversely, the more choice, the higher the monthly premiums and co-payments.

PREMIUMS, DEDUCTIBLES, AND CO-PAYMENTS DEFINED

Premium:
Monthly payment that gives you membership in the plan.

Deductible:
The amount you must pay out of pocket in any given year before plan benefits kick in. There is no deductible for HMOs, or for the HMO part of tiered plans such as a POS. PPOs often impose a deductible.

Copayment:
The amount you fork over at a visit to a doctor, or for a service or hospitalization. HMOs have zero or minimal co-payments. PPOs charge a bigger co-payment. Tiered plans charge a co-payment for all non-HMO visits, and often for an HMO visit that is not to, or preauthorized by, your primary care doctor.

Managed Care: HMOs, PPOs, POSs, and Tiered Plans

These groups compete against each other for patients. Their primary method is to negotiate with employers for contracts with employees. So your employer almost always determines your choice of insurance plans.

You may be presented with one plan only, as a fait accompli. Or you may be offered a choice of plans. This is more likely to be the case when you have a big, rich employer and a big, diverse work force. By diverse, I don't mean race, religion, or gender preference; I mean *money*. The people at the top of the pay-scale hierarchy will probably opt for a PPO, with lots of choice, regardless of the high premiums, deductibles, and co-payments. The workers are more likely to opt for the nearly free but highly restricted care offered by an HMO.

Whether or not your choice is predetermined for you, it is crucial for both your health and your bank account that you understand the rules of the game.

"You can always choose your own primary care provider!" This is often presented as a key benefit. In fact, this is the first decision plans want you to make: "First choose your PCP."

If you are a very low risk patient, that will probably be fine. But if you have any of the risks we've just reviewed, this choice is a poor place to start.

Your own doctor, referred to as your primary care provider (PCP), is the key to all other care: specialists, studies (lab or imaging), second opinions, and hospitalization.

Your insurance company may tell you that a certain specialist, emergency room, hospital, or service is "covered." But that only means that the insurance company has a contract with that entity. If that entity does not have a contract with your PCP's network, medical group, or IPA (independent physician association) it is *not* covered for you.

Gatekeepers

Besides the network factor, which determines *which* specialists and services you can use, there is a gatekeeper factor—your PCP, who may be required to decide *whether* you qualify to make use of a specialist, study, or service within the network. In some plans, that specialist, study, or service will be paid for *only* if you have a formal referral from your PCP.

Moreover, your PCP can't just go around making choices on her own. She has to follow the rules of the medical group. For instance, your PCP may believe that you need to have a mole biopsied and removed by a dermatologist; but the network you and she are embedded in may require that she perform that minor surgery herself.

Many medical groups use the same restrictions that Medicare does, when it comes to a referral. This means that a patient only qualifies if his or her disease state meets Medicare's tests of severity or complexity.

The Alphabet Soup

There are three kinds of managed care, the HMO (health maintenance organization), the PPO (preferred provider organization), and the POS (point of service). They differ as the following chart indicates:

Type of Plan	Role of PCP	Specialist Within Network	Out-of-Network	Deductible	Paper-work
HMO	PCP and gatekeeper	Referral from PCP required	Emergency only, as defined by HMO	No	Done for you
POS	PCP and gatekeeper	Referral from PCP required	Referral from PCP required	For out-of-network referrals	Done for you within network
PPO	PCP only	Self-refer	Self-refer and hefty Copayment	For out-of-network referrals	Done for you within network

HMO (Health Maintenance Organization):
Least Expensive, Fewest Options

You pay a low monthly premium. In return, your HMO provides full service, from preventive care, labs, and imaging studies to specialist care, hospitalization, and medical equipment, such as walkers and wheelchairs, with only minimum co-payments.

High volume and little choice allow the HMO to be very cost efficient.

As one would expect, therefore, the restrictions on HMO patients are very stringent. Your PCP is required to/rewarded for doing many procedures that otherwise might be done by a specialist: casting fractures, sewing up face lacerations, managing severe or complex cases of diabetes, arthritis, and asthma.

Only your PCP can refer you to a specialist or for a service, such as a colonoscopy. You cannot refer yourself.

Moreover, your PCP will have to follow the HMO rules before referring you to a specialist or ordering special equipment, such as a wheelchair, or treatment, such as a bone marrow transplant. Your condition must reach a certain stated level of need before you can be referred, even though these services are "provided within the HMO network."

You cannot go to an out-of-network specialist at all, with or without your PCP's approval, unless you pay for it yourself (or unless you have a truly rare problem, such as a pregnancy with conjoined twins).

A rare exception: True emergencies treated by an out-of-network facility *may* be approved for payment, but the HMO definition of an emergency is usually very narrow. For instance, if you have chest pain but turn out not to have had a heart attack, the HMO might pay for your out-of-network emergency room visit, but is very unlikely to pay for your overnight stay for observation in the hospital.

Finally, there are smaller, powerful networks *within* the HMO, called IPAs. See Part 3, Catching Your Lobster, p. 172.

PPO (Preferred Provider Organization): Most Choice

You pay a fixed monthly premium, and the PPO covers practically all of the cost (except a fairly hefty co-payment) as long as you stay within the services provided by the PPO network. Beyond this, there are three differences between an HMO and a PPO:

- You can go outside the network for specialist services, and the PPO will pay a part of the costs.

- You can see any specialist, inside or out-of-network, without your PCP ordering it, though you will pay extra for doing so. A lot extra, if you choose out-of-network. No prior approval is necessary.

- You may not start to get reimbursed until you have paid enough out-of-pocket to reach a predetermined deductible amount.

Co-payments are likely to be higher than for HMOs.

In a PPO, your primary care provider plays only one role: that of your doctor and advisor. She or he is *not* a gatekeeper. However, it is crucial to check out the rest of the network, including its hospital, emergency room, maternity facilities, and so on. It can be very expensive to go out of network.

POS (Point of Service)

You pay a monthly premium, and the POS provides a network of physicians and services. Like an HMO, if you stay within the network, your co-payments are very low or nonexistent, and there is no deductible to be met. But like a PPO, you are not limited to network providers. However, if you go out of network:

- You must have a referral from your primary care physician.

- There is a deductible that must be met.

- Co-payments for out-of-network care are high.

Tiered Plans

A tiered plan combines an HMO with a PPO. For any given medical occasion, you can opt for no choice and no (or tiny) co-payments, or lots of choice but with a deductible and a high co-payment.

Traps

Bear in mind that each plan also has a policy toward not-quite-medical services. Hardly any managed care plan of any kind will pay for the following: speech therapy, dental/orthodontic work, ordinary vision check ups, ADD evaluations, and kindergarten readiness evaluations. Before you count on such services being covered, read the booklet or call the plan itself.

Watch out for hidden language. For instance, many plans state that they will pay for speech therapy caused by medical problems. However, if the speech problem is caused by early hearing loss due to middle ear infections, or by the pacifier use encouraged by some pediatricians for the first two years of life, they will not pay. From the insurance point of view, speech therapy is covered *only* for congenital deformities or trauma to the mouth and vocal cords. Many will not even pay for speech therapy for children born with hearing loss.

Finally, be wary of other situations that seem to the patient as if they ought to be covered but which may well not be, because they are considered "cosmetic." These include breast reduction surgery, correction of deformed or missing external ears or of a cosmetically deformed skull, use of a plastic surgeon instead of the emergency room surgeon to suture an unsightly laceration, etc.

PART 3: CATCHING YOUR LOBSTER

"I didn't know I couldn't go to my local emergency room anymore! I just got a bill for $1,286, and my plan won't pay it!"

"I was on this same plan for five years, but this year, all of a sudden, it doesn't cover my kids' pediatrician!"

"My insurance contract says that I can see Dr. Famous Specialist, but my own doctor says that I can't—because of something called an IPA! What is an IPA anyway, a grocery store chain or what?"

If the designers of our health care system had sat down with the *intent* of making it a bureaucratic maze studded with traps, they couldn't have been more successful.

A FABLE

(I have put the managed care equivalent in parenthesis and italics.)

You simply adore lobster. You pay $50.00 entrance to a big restaurant that boasts of its lobster dishes. *(You choose an HMO plan that clearly includes your irreplaceable eye surgeon, Dr. Lobster.)* But once you choose your waitperson *(your primary care provider)*, it appears the only meal he can give you is the daily special: scrod, boiled potatoes, and brussels sprouts. *(Eye surgeon Brussels W. Scrod.)*

"Oh No!" you object. "It says right here in the menu, Lobster Thermidor!"

(Bamboozled!)

You are now told that your entrance fee comes with restrictions.

You can have lobster *only* if your waitperson is allowed to serve lobster. And your waitperson is not in the lobster group. He is in the scrod group. *(The primary care provider may only refer within the network, and your irreplaceable surgeon, Dr. Lobster, is not within that network—even though Lobster is contracted with your HMO. In your PCP's network, the eye surgeon is, alas, Dr. Scrod. What you know of Dr. Scrod you do not like.)*

Disgusted, you find a different waitperson, one who is in the lobster group. *(At the monthly opportunity to do so, you opt to change to a primary care provider who is in the same network as irreplaceable Dr. Lobster.)* With a sigh of relief, you order Lobster Thermidor.

Oh no! *This* waitperson also says "No, no lobster for you! The restaurant's management has a preset list of characteristics of customers who are entitled to lobster, and you don't fulfill the requirements." *(Many HMOs have strict requirements having to do with severity of disease to be met before a PCP can refer you to a specialist.)*

You plead with your waitperson to make an exception for you. He says that would cost him a reduced paycheck. You offer to reimburse the missed amount; he says no, it wouldn't just be his paycheck: the paycheck of every waitperson on the staff would be docked, and they'd all be furious. *(The networks in an HMO are called IPAs. These are groups of physicians who contract with the HMO, and receive a chunk of the money you and other patients pay the HMO. The IPA then sets up its own contracts with a subset of specialists. The IPA also imposes rules of care that are more restrictive than the HMO's rules. If one physician in the IPA breaks the rules, the total fund of money is reduced and the whole IPA is "punished.")*

You say that you'll pay cash for the damn lobster yourself. But your waitperson says no, the lobster may not be served to people who don't play by the rules. *(Many HMOs model their restrictions on those of Medicare, and Medicare does not allow patients to "upgrade" their care by paying cash. For instance, if your contract only pays for a partial colonoscopy [halfway up the bowel], you cannot pay the doctor extra to get the whole thing examined.)*

Welcome to scrod and brussels sprouts. It may well be adequate nutrition, but it's not what you had in mind.

Back to Managed Care

Somebody's getting lobster (your one and only specialist, hospital, emergency room)—but not you. Once you have decided upon your choice of primary care provider, you may or may not be "entitled" to the care you thought you were entitled to. The rules aren't posted or written clearly, and loopholes lurk. You can't even buy your way out, most of the time.

If you and your insurance dependents do not, in the coming year, require particular specialists, hospitals, and emergency rooms, then the selection of your PCP is less fraught with worry. Otherwise, common sense would tell you that your specialist, hospital, or emergency room is your first priority, and to choose a plan with that in mind.

However, it is extremely difficult to choose your health plan with special needs in mind *because the insurance plans do not want you to do so.*

If you and everyone else approached this decision in an informed fashion, the whole managed care scheme would come tumbling down. Networks, such as PPOs and medical groups and IPAs would be forced to contract *only* with the highest quality hospitals, emergency rooms, and specialists. Otherwise, nobody would sign up for plans that offered less qualified choices.

But if you can be persuaded that your most important choice is your PCP, your PCP's Network has you at their mercy. (You won't get lobster.)

So don't do it. Instead, start with the "lobster" (the most important specialist, hospital, etc. and work your way back to the choice of "waitperson" (your primary care provider) or even to the choice of restaurant (insurance provider). See chart next page: "Choosing Your Health Care Plan."

Choosing Your Health Care Plan

Step 1→	Step 2 →	Step 3 →	Step 4 →	Step 5 →
Identify Most Crucial Medical Entity ("CME")	**Pull ALL plans that cover CME**	**Decide on HMO vs. PPO vs. POS**	**Each plan: Find the Network that covers your CME**	**Choose your PCP from within that Network.**

For example: Subspecialist:		Factors:	PPO & POS: "Medical	Factors:
· Cardiac		· Cost	Group"	· Reputation
· Cancer		· Covers	HMO:	· Location
· Arthritis		multiple	"IPA"	· Office
· Children's		CMEs		ambience
Specialist				· Languages
				spoken
Hospital:				
· Maternity				
· Children's				
· Cancer				
· University-affiliated				
Emergency Room:				
· Closest				
· Children's				
· Level 3				

PART 4: START AT THE LOBSTER AND
WORK YOUR WAY BACKWARDS

The most important managed care concept to grasp is the concept of the network. A network is a web of physicians, hospitals, emergency rooms, and other services. Each network is contracted to refer patients *only* to other entities on the same network. The network you will be assigned to is the one to which your PCP belongs. This is true whether you have a PPO, POS, or HMO medical plan.

The second most important managed care concept to grasp is that the contract you signed with your insurance plan is not the contract you have with your network. That plan contract is overridden by the contract that your primary care physician has with your network. The network restricts your access to entities on your insurance plan.

For example, your insurance plan (with Aetna, Blue Cross, Prudential, etc.) may state that Dr. Lobster, or The World's Best Hospital, or whatever, is "covered." But this is true *only* if Dr. Lobster or TWBH or whatever is contracted to the network of your PCP.

- Blue Cross is an insurance provider.

  - Prudent Buyer is a Blue Cross PPO network.

- Blue Cross, Aetna, etc. are insurance providers that offer a variety of HMOs.

  - Such HMOs bear names that don't really give much information, such as Pacificare HMO, or Islands HMO, or whatever. They are large networks of providers.

    - Within each HMO network, groups of physicians and facilities are subcontracted. These groups are called IPAs.

- Your choice of IPA is dependent on your choice of primary care provider.
- Exception: Sometimes your employer will choose your HMO *and* your IPA, by assigning you a primary care provider.

Result: the insurance policy may say that a particular person, place or service is covered. However, your PPO network and your HMO network can override this coverage, and deny you access. Moreover, your IPA network overrides the HMO coverage, and denies you even its restricted access. So how do you make sure that your highest priority hospitals, specialists, emergency rooms are "covered" by your Plan?

STRATEGY

Start backwards. List *the lobster* first.

Then examine your choice of insurance companies, types of health care plans, and their networks, to see which ones "cover" those needs.

Choose the health care plan that is both affordable and whose particular network and/or IPA covers the most urgent needs.

Then see which primary care doctors are on that network, and choose one.

PART 5: CHOOSING YOUR OWN PARTICULAR PRIMARY CARE PHYSICIAN

Next time you meet a doctor, and you sit down in his office and he starts to talk, if you have the sense that he isn't listening to you, that he's talking down to you, that he isn't treating you with respect, listen to that feeling. You have thin-sliced him and found him wanting.[28]

---

28. Malcolm Gladwell, *Blink*

However much we long for Marcus Welby, it is less important to know and love your doctor than to trust and respect him. And your prospects may benefit from his treating you with the cool commitment of a professional rather than the comforting warmth of a friend.[29]

Which one is right?

Malcolm Gladwell makes a very confusing judgment about doctors. He says that doctors who are patient-friendly are less likely to be sued, even when they make dire errors, than doctors who come off as disrespectful, arrogant, abrupt, etc., even though those doctors make fewer such errors!

So you'd think that Gladwell would tell us to seek out those doctors with the poor bedside manners, and just bear with them. But no. He gives every indication that the thin-slicing method, the gut feeling about such traits as kindness, humility, humor, is the one to trust.

But then there's the point of view of the *Time* reporters, based apparently on their interviews with numbers of physicians: Go for the cool and distant, and you're likely to get more professional care.

I side with Malcolm Gladwell.

If there is one thing I've learned during Chuck's illness, my own pediatric practice, and the writing of this book, it's this: Kindness, humility, and humor all count hugely. You need a primary care physician who is someone you can talk to, who will listen to you, and who will welcome your on-the-job monitoring of your physicians and reading your own medical record. Such a doctor is much more likely to say "I don't know,"

---

29. Nancy Gibbs and Amanda Bower, "Q: What Scares Doctors? A: Being the Patient; What Insiders Know About Our Health-Care System That the Rest of Us Need to Learn," *Time* magazine, May 1, 2006, page 48

or "I hadn't noticed that." Because such a doctor cares more for the patient than for his ego.

Trusting Your Instincts

Here I am, a primary care physician for decades. I feel like, and often am treated as, a member of my young patients' extended families. When Chuck was sick, they sent me drawings and cards, prayers and kind thoughts. When I returned to practice after his death, they patted me and didn't expect me to laugh much. When I started to be able to laugh, they noticed, and told me that they'd noticed. I have been so lucky.

During these years, I have had to suggest to several patients that they transfer to a different pediatrician, one with affiliations with a different medical group or network or IPA.

In one case, it was an eight-year-old with a devastating genetic neurological disease. He needed a custom made, power-operated wheelchair with restraints. Not only was he easily exhausted and uncoordinated, he was unable to hear and understand. He'd head out into the street, or kick a passerby. Moreover, he weighed more than eighty pounds because of the medications he was taking. When he lay down and refused to move, his parents couldn't pick him up, much less carry him. The family literally couldn't leave the house.

The Medical Group of which I was a member denied the costly wheelchair. They were using Medicare guidelines, which stated that no one could get a wheelchair unless they were so immobilized they needed it to get to the bathroom.

My senior partner and I were outraged.

We said, "But he's only eight." We said, "Besides, if that's the criterion for a wheelchair, wouldn't it be cheaper to get a bedpan?"

We were reminded many times that the multithousand dollar wheelchair would cost not just us and our practice, but the entire medical group. My physician colleagues in the Group would have their own paychecks dented by our demands.

We finally got the wheelchair, but the process was so contentious and exhausting, the parents found a primary care physician on, I hope, a more accommodating IPA.

I use this as an illustration because it brings up something nobody wants to look at. There is a true conflict of interest for the physician. But it's not just the doctor's paycheck versus the patient's need. It's the *colleagues'* paychecks versus the patient's need, with the PCP getting the worst of all worlds. The patient and family are angry and frustrated by the delay in getting the wheelchair. The medical group feels betrayed by the PCP who has broken the rules.

So you need a PCP who can deal with these issues, and help you as much as possible.

My suggestion:

- Use the list of primary care providers that you now know are in the same network or IPA as your "lobster"—your most crucial medical priority.

- Then make an appointment for your annual check-up or a non-serious symptom. Think of it partly as a trial run, to check out the office and the individual PCP.

- A week or so later, ask for your medical record from that visit, and judge the doctor's accuracy, completeness, and clarity. Think about how you felt after the appointment.

- If you sense a bad aura, don't assume that this is a fixed quality of the doctor; it may be a natural response to something that has happened that you can't even guess. Give one or two more tries.

- If the chemistry just isn't right, you can switch PCPs—usually at the beginning of the month. Just make sure that your new one is from the same "short list" that includes your "lobster."

I wish you a mutually trusting, long-term, fulfilling dialogue with your primary care provider, and your entire network.

Glossary

Authorization: Permission to obtain a service or treatment so that insurance will pay for it. If you get permission ahead of time, it's called "prior authorization." If you try to get a service or treatment paid for after it's been performed, it's called "retroactive authorization."

Benefit: A service that your particular version of your insurance company is prepared to pay for, within their stated restrictions

Benign: Substitute "not cancer" or "not the dangerous form"

Catheter: Substitute "tube." Catheters can be inserted just about anywhere in the body, for just about any function—from removing a quarter from a child's breathing tube, to carrying chemotherapy into a large blood vessel, to providing a convenient exit for urine.

Covered: An entity that your particular version of your insurance plan will pay for, in whole or in part, as long as you stay in your network and obtain prior **authorization**

Clinician or Clinical Physician: A doctor who interacts with the patient, makes decisions about diagnosis, orders studies and treatments

Cosmetic: A problem or treatment whose only effect is aesthetic (having to do with appearance). Cosmetic treatments usually are not covered by insurance. Each Plan has its own definition of cosmetic. For instance, if a baby is born without ears, that may be considered a cosmetic problem. But if its hearing mechanisms do not work, that is considered **functional** because the ability to hear is a normal ability. So the hearing problem itself may receive covered benefits.

Data Doctor: A physician whose specialty consists of interpreting studies. Examples: radiologist, pathologist.

DIAGNOSTIC REASONING

Doctors make most diagnoses using a skill we're all familiar with: pattern recognition. That is, match the "picture" of your patient on the exam table with all the "pictures" in your long-term memory, and find one that matches as closely as possible.

Clearly, the more pictures the physician has accumulated, and the more efficient the matching process, the better the chance of an accurate diagnosis.

There are three flaws inherent to this system:

1. Doctors are trained to follow the dictum that "When you hear hoof beats, think of horses." That is, when you are matching up your patient, limit your possible patterns to the most common entities, not the exotic ones: no zebras, wildebeests, or unicorns, please. This is fine, except when the pictures don't quite match. Then you'd better consider just about anything with hoofs. If it doesn't look like a typical case of chicken pox, you'd better eliminate smallpox as a possibility, no matter how unlikely it seems.

2. Doctors have access only to the experiences they have filed in their long-term memories. Young doctors struggle to enlarge

that fund, and older doctors struggle to extract those memories in the face of "senior moments."

3. Doctors often don't know what they don't know. I may think I know how to evaluate an injured ankle, but suppose I missed the part about asking my patient to try to stand on tiptoe. Well, I am sure to be surprised when two weeks later, he turns out to have a permanent limp from the ruptured Achilles tendon I failed to diagnose.

One solution to this problem is the use of algorithms, or "decision trees." A decision tree starts with a symptom, physical finding, or data abnormality. At every "branch" in the "tree," a question is asked. The answer guides you to another branch, and so on, until you arrive at the most likely diagnosis.

The problem, of course, is deciding which symptom, finding, or abnormality to start with.

A solution to this problem generally has to involve computers. Jason Maude founded a company to come up with such a solution, which he named Isabelle Healthcare, after his daughter. When Isabelle was a young child, she came very close to dying of a complication of chicken pox that went unrecognized by her doctors. As reported in the *New York Times* (February 22, 2006, p. C4) by columnist David Leonhardt, Isabelle is a special kind of software. It "allows doctors to type in a patient's symptoms and, in response, spits out a list of possible causes. It does not replace doctors, but makes sure they can consider some unobvious possibilities."

The service costs $80,000 a year for a typical hospital and $750 a year for an individual doctor.

Endoscopy: A tube with a fiber-optic light and a teeny camera is threaded into a body opening, such as nose, throat, intestine, windpipe, to see what is going on and record it on film

Etiology: (eet-ee-OL-uh-jee) Substitute "cause"

Functional: Substitute "normal." May also be used by insurance companies to define coverage; see **cosmetic.**

General Practitioner: A physician whose practice is open to a broad range of patients, defined by age or other general category. From this group is chosen your PCP (primary care provider). Examples:

Family Practitioner: can treat most problems of all ages and both sexes

Internist: can treat most problems of adults

Pediatrician: can treat most problems of children and teenagers

General Surgeon: can treat most surgical conditions

Obstetrician: can treat most pregnancies

Orthopedic surgeon or *Orthopod*: can treat most bone and joint problems

GYN or *gynecologist*: can treat pregnancy and delivery, and most problems arising in female organs

Gross: Substitute "big" or "large" or "large amount"

Grossly: How it appears to the naked eye, as in "grossly normal"—as opposed to how it looks under the microscope, or when subjected to lab tests

Group or Medical Group: The network of physicians, hospitals, and facilities in which a primary care provider is embedded, within which you will receive the most covered benefits. If you are in an HMO (see Appendix), your group is called an IPA (independent physicians' association). If you are in a PPO (see Appendix), your group is the PPO network.

Imaging Procedures: Any procedure that takes a picture of body parts or functions

Contrast: a substance is given by mouth or by catheter (into an artery, vein, the bladder, etc.) to give greater accuracy to the imaging study by outlining or filling an organ or vessel

CT or *CAT:* Computed Tomography scan, where the X ray camera takes lots of views and the computer puts them together into a three-dimensional picture

Echocardiogram: ultrasound (see below) of the heart and vessels

Fluoroscopy: the X ray camera serves as a movie camera, catching quick images of a body part in motion

MRI: Magnetic Resonance Imaging, in which a giant magnet acts on the electric charges in your body's cells to magically make a picture, especially of soft tissues

Nuclear scan: very low-intensity radioactive substance is given instead of the usual contrast material. The imaging study locates the nuclear material where it is most concentrated.

Plain film: you hold still and the X ray camera snaps a "photo" of your innards

Ultrasound: radar, with sound waves bouncing off tissues, forms an image that can record movement, as of a fetus, or of the heart

Invasive: A procedure or treatment that involves "invading" the integrity of the body, such as by incision or insertion. Needles, tubes, and general anesthesia are considered invasive. **Noninvasive** means that the integrity of the body is not invaded; but this doesn't mean it doesn't upset the patient: try giving a child nose drops.

Lesion: Substitute "possible cancer or other bad thing"

Malignant: Two meanings: 1. Cancer 2. A dire form of something, as in "malignant fever"

Mass: Substitute "possible cancer"

Metastasis: (met-ASS-tuh-sis) Substitute "spread of cancer"; also **metastatic** (met-uh-STAT-ic): malignant tumors that have spread from original site to elsewhere

Negative: Substitute "normal"

Pathologic: Substitute "abnormal"

Positive: substitute "abnormal," unless it describes a pregnancy test, in which case substitute "pregnant"

Progressive: Likely to get worse

Non-progressive: Not likely to change in either direction

Radiology: See **Imaging procedures**

Septic: Overwhelmingly infected

Sign: Objective evidence of something: as opposed to **symptom**, which is a sensation experienced, or which seems to be experienced, by the patient

Specialist: A physician who is not a primary care doctor. This includes three levels of training:

1. Physicians who have taken their primary residency, and are board certified, in a field that narrows their range of patients, ophthalmology, for instance

2. Physicians who have taken a primary residency in which they are board certified, plus a secondary residency which focuses on an even smaller group of patients, *pediatric* ophthalmology, for instance

3. Physicians who, after their secondary residency, take yet another one to focus even more narrowly, such as a pediatric retinal specialist. I do not know where this will end, nor do I know exactly how to refer to these folks—superspecialists or sub-subspecialists. To find out more, go to the American Board of Medical Specialties at **www.abms.org**.

Specialties: You can usually figure out what the specialty and specialist are called by looking at the word describing what or whom they deal with:

Arthro: joints

Cardio: the heart

Derm: the skin

Gastro: the entire gut, throat to anus

Geriatric: older people

Gyn: female organs

Heme, hema, hemato: blood

Immuno: immune system

Laryngo: mouth and throat

Neonatal: new babies

Neuro: the brain, spinal cord, and nerves

Onco: cancer

Ophthal: eye

Ortho: bones and joints

Oto: ear, hearing

Pediatric: children with a specific problem. (pediatric cardiologist, pediatric surgeon, etc.)

Perinatal: fetuses

Procto: rectum

Pulmo: lungs

Thoracic: chest

Uro: urinary tract system, both sexes

Toxic: Dangerously ill

Unremarkable: Substitute "seems normal" (do not confuse this term with a put-down)

MINIGLOSSARY OF MEDICAL ABBREVIATIONS
YOU MAY SEE IN YOUR CHART

DOL: Day of Life (found in newborn charts)

EDC: Estimated Date of Confinement (!); predicted date of birth

ENT: Ear, Nose, and Throat specialist; fancy term: otolaryngologist or otorhinolaryngologist

HAV: The Hepatitis A virus, which you can get from contaminated food and water. There is a very effective vaccine.

HBV: The Hepatitis B virus, spread mostly but not entirely by sex and needles, including blood transfusion. There is a very effective vaccine for this dangerous illness, most effective when given to young children.

HCV: The Hepatitis C virus. There is no vaccine as yet for this viral cause of serious liver disease; the virus is passed by blood transfusions, dirty needles, and sex.

Hib: Hemophilus influenza type B: A very dangerous kind of bacteria, especially for children. It can cause meningitis, pneumonia, and a dangerous, rapidly fatal swelling of the airway. The very effective vaccine should be given to all babies, starting at 2 months of age.

HIV: The AIDS virus. There is no vaccine as yet.

HPV: Human papilloma virus, which is passed sexually and is the cause of a high proportion of cervical cancer (cancer of the neck of the womb). There is a highly effective vaccine, recommended for preteens and teenagers but it will not protect someone who has already contracted it.

NAD: In No Acute Distress; not having severe or sharp pain

NPO: Nothing By Mouth

OU: Both eyes; OD is right eye and OS is left eye

PO: By Mouth

PR: By Rectum; suppository

R/O: Rule Out

SOB: Shortness of Breath

WD/WN: Well developed; Well Nourished

Index